The #1 Ketogenic Intermittent Fasting Diet Book

A Step-by-Step Guide to Keto, Ketosis, Fasting, Weight Loss, Building Lean Muscle, and Low-Carb High-Fat High-Protein Meal Plans

Table of Contents

Introduction 5
Chapter 1: The Keto Diet and the Body's Reaction to it 8
    What is the Keto Diet? 8
    The Keto Diet's Weight Loss Results 11
    The Trouble with Carbohydrates 16
    The Trouble with Sugar 18
    What about Cholesterol? 20
    How Your Metabolism Works 22
    How Keto Balances Your Hormones 24

Chapter 2: How to Follow the Keto Diet 27
    Fats and Carbs on the Keto Diet 27
    Ready for Keto? 29
    A Balanced Keto Diet 31

Chapter 3: Keto Meal Plans 37
    Meal Plans 37
        BREAKFAST 39
        LUNCH 45
        DINNER 50
    What are Fat Bombs? 61
        SWEET FAT BOMBS 63
        SAVORY FAT BOMBS 70

Chapter 4: The Keto Flu 78
    What is the Keto Flu? 78
    Why Do We Get the Keto Flu? 80
    How to Fight the Keto Flu 82

Chapter 5: Exercising on a Keto Diet **88**
   Exercising on Keto 88
   Pre and Post Workout 95
   Smoothie Recipes 99

Chapter 6: Tips to Get You Started & Mistakes to Avoid! **101**
   Tips to Embrace a Keto Lifestyle 101
   Common Mistakes on a Keto Diet 105
   Motivational Work Out Tips! 108

Chapter 7: Intermittent Fasting **111**
   What is Intermittent Fasting? 111
   The Health Benefits of Fasting 113
   Solving the Misconception about Fasting 117
   How to Get Started 121

Conclusion **126**

Introduction

Congratulations on downloading The #1 Ketogenic Intermittent Fasting Diet Book: *A Step by Step Guide to Keto, Ketosis, Fasting, Weight Loss, Building Lean Muscle, and Low-Carb High-Fat High-Protein Meal Plans.* If you've downloaded this book, chances are, you are curious about the keto diet that you've been hearing so much about. This diet has become very popular in recent years because of the weight loss results it produces and the positive effects on overall health. It does more than just help you drop those stubborn pounds — it can even lower your blood pressure, regulate your blood sugar levels, and balance your hormone levels! The goal of this diet is to change the types of foods you're eating to push your body away from burning carbohydrates for energy and using the fat molecules your body has stored away. That's right — the energy is already there! Your body has saved it away as a backup source, but as you're eating carbohydrates throughout the body, the body keeps using those carbs instead. Changing your diet so you're eating more high-quality fats means the body will not have a carbohydrate intake to use for energy, so it will burn ketone molecules made out of the fat you have already stored. That means you will lose weight!

To follow a keto diet, your daily count of nutrients should come from 75% fat, 20% protein, and ~5% carbohydrates. Now, the diet can be tweaked a little if you're an athlete and need more carbs before a workout. Or you can do a cyclical diet where you rotate throughout the week and have a few carb-eating days to renew your energy. It can seem overwhelming at first trying to learn about this new diet and making these lifestyle changes. This book is here to help! We have a preparation list on how to help you approach a keto diet. That begins with cleaning out your pantry and getting rid of those tempting carbs! Then you will need to shop and stock up on keto-friendly ingredients to prepare your meals.

People often think of a diet as restricting. And yes, you're cutting out carbs and sugars, but the keto diet has a rich area of protein, dairy, fruits, and vegetables that you can choose from! You can even have keto-friendly dark chocolates as long it contains a content of 80% or higher cacao! If you're struggling, we have more than 30 recipes to help you make keto-friendly breakfast, lunch, and dinner meals! Not to mention, another list of meal ideas and snacks that you can have! With this information, you are ready to meal plan and prepare food on a keto diet so you are getting the nutrients you need. We even provided you with recipes for more than 20+ keto fat bombs! These can be sweet or savory snacks with a high-fat content and low carbs that can be used as a meal substitute or as a snack to up your macro count. They are easy to make and need simple ingredients that you probably have on hand already!

If you've seen someone start the keto diet, you maybe recall them having a few weeks where their body needed to adjust. That period is often called the "keto flu" because it has flu-like symptoms such as weakness, dizziness, difficulty sleeping, stomach pains, or muscle cramps. That can sound intense but keep in mind what you are trying to do! You have to change the pathway of how your body burns energy from using carbs to using ketones. It's natural that it will need a few weeks to adjust. We will give you some tips on how to fight the keto flu and adjust quickly to the keto diet! Once you're over that period, you will be pleasantly surprised to see your body has adjusted and you're shedding water weight!

Another important part of the keto diet is exercising. It is good for your overall health but it can also help you lose weight faster! For some high-intensity workouts, your performance could be impaired on a keto diet. That's because when you're playing sports like rugby or soccer that do not have frequent breaks, your body will need instant energy from carb sources and it won't find any if you're on a keto diet. Same with heavy weight lifting or long-distance running or swimming. But the keto diet encourages you to include some light physical activities in your day. We will give you some tips on how to start, what activities to do, and what activities to abstain from when it comes to your health. If you're an athlete, we even list some keto-friendly protein supplement powders you can use in your pre-workout smoothies! With a list of supplements and the recommended usage as well as a list of smoothie recipes, you are ready to work out and to ensure you are getting the most out of your keto diet!

Maybe you want to try fasting to get rid of the weight. You'll be surprised to know intermittent fasting (or fasting in on-and-off blocks of time) actually has a ton of health benefits too! Not only will it help you lose weight, but it can lower your cholesterol and blood sugar, reboot your immune system, and even delay signs of aging! It can seem counterintuitive that going without food can actually help you live longer — but you'll see how the research proves it! Not only that, we debunk some misconceptions about fasting and help you get started on easy beginner's models that you don't even realize you may be following!

If you're nervous or hesitant about starting the keto diet or intermittent fasting, then this is the perfect book to give you the information you need! We also have a list of tips to get you started and a list of mistakes that you should avoid. Packed with keto-friendly recipes, this is the book to get you started on a healthier lifestyle today!

Chapter 1:

The Keto Diet and the Body's Reaction to it

What is the Keto Diet?

The ketogenic or the keto diet for short is a popular diet that has become a national phenomenon because of the weight loss and overall health benefits it produces! This is a diet low in carbohydrates that urges the body into a state called "ketosis". Ketosis is when the body's liver produces ketones to be used as energy instead of glucose that is produced when the body is on a normal carbohydrates diet. When you eat something high in carbohydrates, the body's first pathway to produce energy is to produce glucose or sugar molecules as an energy source. Glucose is the easiest molecule to make so the body takes that route first! Insulin processes the glucose in the bloodstream and takes it around the body. That's why an increase in carbohydrates can lead to an increase in insulin in the body which can dramatically raise your blood sugar. If the body is making glucose to power you through the day, the fat molecules you have stored are not being used! What a keto diet does is lower the amount of carbohydrates so that the body enters the state of ketosis to burn stored fat molecules instead. Ketones are what the body produces in the liver by burning the stored fat molecules and using that for fuel.

Some people criticize the keto diet for saying it's unnaturally pushing the body towards ketosis. But that's not true at all! Our bodies are designed with multiple routes to make energy to adapt in changing environments. The only reason your body produces glucose first is that it's the easiest and convenient way to process those carbohydrates into energy molecules. That's what you've gotten used to! If you slowly take away carbohydrates and maintain a low carb diet, the body will begin to enter ketosis and burn ketones as the primary energy source. That means all that stubborn fat that you haven't been able to get rid of will finally be used and you'll shed pounds! The state of ketosis and minimizing carbohydrates offers many health benefits including weight loss, reducing the chances of having Type 2 diabetes, and overall acute mental health.

So what is the breakdown of a keto diet? A standard keto diet works to keep the carb intake at a minimum and the fat intake at a maximum! Protein works in the middle to provide you the calories and energy you need.

75% fat
20% protein
~5% carbohydrates

There are other types of the keto diet which can work in rotating days. The cyclical ketogenic diet (CKD) has 5 keto days and then 2 high-carbohydrate days. That might not be as effective to help you lose weight and gain the health benefits, but it's a great start to people who want to embrace the diet but can't make a full-time commitment. The targeted ketogenic diet (TKD) has some leniency and lets you add carbohydrates around workouts. These methods are more commonly used by athletes or weightlifters who are struggling to maintain their caloric count and need a higher carbohydrates intake. A high protein ketogenic diet is similar to the standard one but it ups the protein count. It might look more like 60% fat, 35% protein, and 5% carbs. It is important to note that the standard keto diet is the version most people are familiar with and is the most researched one. When we go on further to speak of the overall health benefits associated with the keto diet, we will be speaking about research based on the standard keto diet.

The Keto Diet's Weight Loss Results

The test groups have been studied and the results are in. The keto diet is an effective way to lose weight and increase your overall health in general! It's been shown that this diet is a better way to lose weight than the low-fat diet. Studies across the globe have shown almost 3 times more weight loss in ketogenic diet test groups than ones on a different diet. The diet also lowered their risk factors for other diseases, lowered the HDL or "bad" cholesterol levels, and reduced the risk of Type 2 diabetes.

What do some of the research say about the ketogenic diet being more helpful with weight loss? Here we have it!

- A 2008 study at Duke University (North Carolina, USA) found that in a group of 84 volunteers with obesity and Type 2 diabetes, the group that was on the low carb ketogenic diet had greater weight loss, losing nearly 11 pounds versus the reduced calorie test group that lost 6 pounds. The ketogenic diet group also improved their blood count, lowered their HDL cholesterol, and improved their fasting glucose numbers. Diabetes medications were either reduced or eliminated in 95% of the low carbohydrate ketogenic diet test group!

- A 2013 study at the University of Melbourne (Melbourne, Australia) conducted an experiment regarding weight regain after being on a keto diet. 39 individuals have completed ketogenic diet for 8 weeks and then reintroduction of foods for 2 weeks. During the keto diet, the test group lost about 13% of body weight. After reintroduction of foods, their appetites, amylin, and leptin levels were lower. This shows that the successful adaptation of the ketogenic diet changes the concentration of hormones in the body to suppress your appetite!

- A 2008 study at Rowett Research Institute (Aberdeen, United Kingdom) found that a low carb diet was more successful in reducing hunger and lowering food intake than other medium carbohydrate non-ketogenic diets. In a study group of obese men, the study group with the low carb diet lost nearly 6.5 kilograms of weight on average than the medium carb group that lost 4.3 kilograms. They also reported their hunger appetite felt lower.

- A 2007 study at Churchill Hospital (Oxford, United Kingdom) found that a group of Type 2 diabetes subjects following a low carbohydrate ketogenic diet had nearly 6.9 kilograms of weight loss compared to the normal diet group which had an average of 2.1 kilograms weight loss. The diet was effective in both the group with and without diabetes.

- A 2009 study on rat test subjects conducted at Case Western Reserve University (Cleveland, Ohio) found that out of test subjects on a fasting, prolonged starvation, or a ketogenic diet, the ketogenic diet group had decreased glucose levels in the cortex and cerebellum of the brain. This data indicates that going through the process of ketosis to harness energy can lower glucose levels in the bloodstream. Rats were imaged in a rodent PET scanner and samples of blood were taken!

There are many, many more studies that have been conducted to show how test subjects on a ketogenic diet had increased weight loss than other diet counterparts. The ketogenic diet has swept the nation because of the weight loss results it produces without the need to count calories or fast for days. This is a diet that produces results and helps you get rid of the weight you haven't been able to shake off!

For your body to lose weight, it's not as simple as just cutting carbs. Your body has to be in the state of ketosis for it to run on ketones in lieu of carbohydrates. If you are not on this state, then you won't lose the fat you already have.

How can you push your body towards weight loss while on this diet? Here are some tips on how the process starts!

Calculate your keto macros. To successfully live by the keto lifestyle, you need to take a look at your macro intake — carbohydrates, protein, and fats. To guide your body towards a state of ketosis, you have to be sure you are following the right ratio of macros. If there are too much carbs, then it won't work. If your protein count is too high, it won't work. You have to try your best to stick to the ketogenic ratio: 75% fat, 20% protein, ~5% carbohydrates! There are many keto calculator apps you can use or find a website online to do the math for you. By keeping a steady count of your diet in the beginning, you can adjust your intake as necessary. If you see you need to further adjust your macros, you can!

Give your body time. Ketosis is a process that takes anywhere from 2 to 7 days depending on each person's body and metabolism. Don't rush it or become impatient if you don't see instant results. This can be especially tough if you're feeling hungry! It's only when your body reaches ketosis that you will see weight loss occur.

Eat a healthy ketogenic diet. Focus on the quality of the keto foods you are eating as you follow the diet. Make sure your dairy and meat products are organic and grass-fed so you are not ingesting any possible steroids or GMOs. Have quality ingredients like fresh lettuce, leafy greens, ghee, avocado, and organic butters.

Exercise! You will definitely lose weight rapidly by adding some physical activity to your day. This is especially true when you're coupling the activity with a keto diet. It doesn't mean you have to become a gym rat and dedicate an hour daily to working out, but you want to make changes so you're more active. Take a short walk around the neighborhood on your way home or take a longer route to get your morning coffee. Make use of the stairs rather than using the lift next time and get off one stop early on the subway to have a few minutes extra walk home. These can be small changes, but they burn calories and those calories add up.

Typically, people starting the keto diet will have a fast water weight loss in the first two weeks anywhere from **2 to 10 pounds**. That's when the keto diet is flushing out the body's water weight because of the reduced carbohydrates consumption. You are not losing fats yet, but it is an indication that the body is in its way to the state of ketosis by first burning reserve glycogen molecules it had. After this initial stage, you might see a more consistent weight loss of **1 to 3 pounds a week** depending on how active you are. If you regularly exercise and go to the gym, you may shed more pounds! One study found that obese patients after being on the ketogenic diet for 2 months shed about 30 pounds in total. By the end of the study, almost 90% of the patients lost at least 10% of their initial weight. You can lose the most weight for the first few months of the diet, but it can be sustained as long as you follow the diet and couple it with an exercise routine that works for you. While getting closer to the desired weight that you want, the weight loss slows down naturally due to the body needing fewer calories.

The Trouble with Carbohydrates

Carbohydrates are a necessary food group and tend to make up nearly half of our daily caloric requirement. They are a great source of energy and they produce most of the glucose moles that our body harnesses as a fuel source to get us through the day. They are burned first for energy after a workout session! But the problem occurs when people have a diet that's too high in carbohydrates. That produces unhealthy side effects and can impact your overall health. Not to mention increase weight gain!

That's because the body stores carbohydrates as fat molecules. This becomes a toxic cyclical process. You might be working out to try and lose weight but if you are eating too many carbohydrates, your body is just continuing to store new fat. This will not help you with your ultimate goal of losing weight. You need a balance in your diet to urge your body to lose the extra fat it has stored away. That's where the keto diet comes in! By having a low amount of carbohydrates, the body is urged into ketosis and produces ketones from your stored fat reserves. That burns up those fat molecules instead of storing new ones!

Another downside of too much carbohydrates is that it increases the level of triglycerides in your blood. These molecules are a type of unhealthy fat molecules that are found in the bloodstream. They are linked to a higher rate of heart disease and can increase your risk of blood clots, swollen arteries, and even a heart attack. When your triglyceride count increases due to a high carb intake, the "good" cholesterol in your body also decreases. More often than not, carbohydrates rich foods are also rich in fat which means your artery walls thicken due to the fat intake. This makes it harder for your body to bump blow and increases your chances for blood clots, or a heart attack, or stroke. By reducing and managing a low consumption of carbohydrates, you can effectively decrease the level of triglycerides in the blood.

High carbohydrate intake is a worrying factor for people who live with Type 2 diabetes. When a person with diabetes or diabetes risk factors has an increased intake of carbohydrates, the body uses insulin to convert these glucose molecules into "storage" molecules for later use. It causes your blood sugar levels to go into overdrive and the body's insulin production system goes haywire at the change of concentration in the blood. By maintaining a diet low in carbohydrates, the body's insulin levels remain more stable which reduce the risk of diabetes in patients who may be at risk. Studies have found that patients who already have Type 2 diabetes can lower their blood sugar and even reduce the medication they take to manage their sugar levels!

The Trouble with Sugar

As we mentioned in the previous section about carbohydrates, the body creates glucose molecules out of the carbs we eat as food. What is glucose? It's a type of simple sugar! When there's an unstable amount of sugar in our bloodstream, it can leave you experiencing mood swings or headaches. You can get false hunger pangs and feel hungry and end up overeating and gaining weight. Fructose sugar fools your metabolism into thinking you aren't full and your body begins to produce more of the hunger hormone. You begin to eat more even though you've had enough! That's why overeating is common if you are not eating a healthy diet where you are limiting your carbs intake and having too much sugar. It's addicting for a reason!

Sugar even increases the level of hormones in your body! When you eat a sugary snack, the body releases a large amount of stress hormones called cortisol to try and stabilize your blood sugar. The body becomes frantic at the hormone rush and it can make you feel irritable or anxious. That's what might bring on mood swings or leave you feeling "sluggish" after a sugary snack.

Foods that are high in sugars can lead to higher chances of getting diabetes, heart disease, and obesity. This is the reason why there's the glycemic scale that measures where foods fall depending on how quickly they affect the blood sugar in the body. High glycemic foods quickly raise your blood sugar. These are the ones patients with diabetes should stay away from. When your body's blood sugar suddenly changes when you eat these foods, your system becomes stressed. It struggles to keep up and manage the sugar level which is when it causes a rush of hormones. Low glycemic foods are ones that keep the blood sugar stable and allow you to feel full longer. Apples, oranges, and cherries are fruits that are low on the glycemic scale. They are naturally sweet foods, but they don't surprise the body with a high intake of sugar at once to cause distress. If you're at risk of diabetes or have diabetes, you've probably been given a list of what foods and fruits are better for you to eat to prevent your blood sugar from increasing dramatically. That can cause headaches, dizziness, or fatigue.

Fruits and vegetables that have natural sugars are better for you than the high fructose corn syrup and processed foods that we are bombarded by on a daily basis. They're the real culprits! This sugar is highly processed! But because it is so much cheaper to produce, many beverage and food companies use it in their products. It's at least 20% sweeter than regular granulated sugar! Be sure you read the label before trying new foods or drinks so you have an idea of how many grams of corn syrup there is per serving!

The most dangerous thing that sugar does is taking you away from having a balanced diet of healthy nutrients and minerals your body needs. A study at the Department of Agriculture determined that people who have a higher concentration of sugar intake in their diet have lower concentrations of vitamins A, B-12, C, and calcium. This is especially dangerous when it comes to young children and teenagers who need a diet full of variety to obtain those common minerals and vitamins. If your diet is filled with unnecessary extra carbs and unhealthy sugars, then you're missing out on eating things that your body actually needs to help you get through puberty, lose weight and gain muscle, and gain overall health benefits.

What about Cholesterol?

When we've mentioned the effects that carbohydrates and sugars have on your health, you've seen the term "good" and "bad" cholesterol mentioned. What is cholesterol exactly? It's a type of fat in the body that stays primarily in the bloodstream. But if there's too much of it, it begins to clog your blood vessels which can lead to serious health problems. This may increase the chances of having a stroke or heart attack.

Cholesterol is naturally produced by the liver, but you can also gain cholesterol from the types of foods that you eat. Foods that are mentioned as high in cholesterol are the culprits for raising your levels. But there are also foods that can raise your "good" cholesterol levels! A healthy diet with variety is important if you want a healthy cholesterol level. As we've mentioned, there are two parts to cholesterol: the low-density lipoprotein cholesterol (LDL) or the "bad" cholesterol which can stick to the blood vessels to cause blockages and the high density lipoprotein (HDL) which is the "good" cholesterol that carries cholesterol back to the liver to break it down.

So how do carbohydrates and sugars impact your cholesterol level? A 2010 study found that people who ate more sugar had lower "good" cholesterol or HDL levels. They had higher levels of triglyceride fat molecules that circulated dangerously in their bloodstream. These molecules store extra energy for the body but they can damage the walls of your arteries and cause blockages in your blood flow. According to the Mayo Health Clinic, you're more likely to have a higher level of triglycerides if you eat a diet composed of high fat, sugar, or alcohol content and if you're not burning off all the energy you consume. In order to lose weight, you have to have a calorie deficit diet which means burning more than you're taking in.

Another way that cholesterol is connected is when it comes to your blood sugar. After you eat carbohydrates and your blood sugar goes up, your body produces insulin to begin storing the glucose as energy. But with an excess of sugar in the blood, the body stores the sugar molecules as LDL molecules instead or the "bad" cholesterol. This is the kind that can lead to damage in your artery walls and increase your risk of having a stroke or heart attack. So, a high carbohydrate diet can lead to an increase in your LDL cholesterol levels.

Sugars that occur naturally like in fruits and vegetables tend to have a different effect on the body's system. They are absorbed more slowly so the body's insulin levels stay stable and levels aren't thrown into shock by a sweet treat. Knowing where a food falls on the glycemic scale can help patients at risk of diabetes make smarter food decisions. Be sure to read the labels before trying new foods so you're aware of the carbohydrate and sugar intake. This will allow you to make a more informed decision as you follow your keto diet!

How Your Metabolism Works

When we talk about the keto diet and about losing weight, we have to talk about how our metabolic system works to produce energy out of the foods we eat. Metabolism is a complex process that describes the process of how the body creates energy out of the food we eat for all our living cellular processes. If people aren't losing weight, they often blame their metabolic system for failing them but it is more complex than that. Other factors like your age, sex, and body size all play a role in your metabolic rate. These differences are normal that occur based on every person's individual makeup.

The problem with fad diets is that they try and severely restrict your calorie intake in hopes that you increase your metabolic rate. But that actually does the opposite! When you're depriving your body of food and limiting the amount of calories you take in, your body stores every single calorie it can when you do eat. Only eating one giant meal doesn't help you lose weight. You want to spread out your meals so that you can burn off the calories with physical activity throughout the day.

Sleep deprivation can also be detrimental to weight loss. If you're not getting enough sleep, your body actually produces an excess of insulin which means you're storing more fat molecules. Rest is important to regulate your body so be sure you're trying to get at least 7 to 9 hours a night or however many hours you need to feel well rested.

Another factor that impacts your metabolism is whether or not you were overweight before and have already had significant weight loss. Researchers theorize that after you lose weight, the shift in your hormones can slow your metabolism and make you feel hungrier even when you aren't. Sometimes you can get medication to help with this sensation so you are not in danger of overeating. But it is a factor in people who have already lost a significant amount of weight and are trying to keep it off. For these people, it's very important that they keep track of their caloric intake so they are not regaining the weight.

The simple matter is the problem occurs when you're eating more calories than you're consuming. With the calories you have left over, your body uses that excess food intake and stores it as fat molecules. To lose weight, you need to have a balance of a healthy diet and staying active to burn off calories. By keeping track of your calorie intake, you are ensuring you are eating healthy foods and then coupling that with burning off any excess energy with exercise.

The keto diet capitalizes on eating the right foods to give you a fulfilled sensation. By eating more healthy fats and protein, the body is burning from the fat reserves it has stored instead of producing new energy molecules. With a healthy meal plan and a combination of steady exercise, the keto diet produces weight loss results and improves overall health.

If you feel that there is a problem with your metabolism or notice troubling trends in your weight gain, it is important you speak with your doctor. You could have a possible thyroid problem or problem with your pituitary gland that is slowing down your metabolism. If you feel dizziness, fatigue, or have severe constipation when starting the diet, you should talk to your doctor. If you have struggled with a history of eating disorders, you should speak to your doctor before making any changes to your meal plan.

How Keto Balances Your Hormones

There is some misinformation out there that states that the keto diet can cause a hormone imbalance. In fact, most of the research states that the keto diet is a great way to balance your hormone levels especially when it comes to regulating insulin levels in diabetes or patients at risk of diabetes. Insulin is produced naturally by the pancreas as the body processes carbohydrates and creates glucose molecules for energy. Most diet fads have a high number of carbohydrates intake which increases a person's blood sugar. That can cause insulin resistance as the body is unable to cope with the constant high blood sugar levels.

But the keto diet does the opposite! It minimizes your carbohydrates intake so your blood sugar is regulated and your body maintains a normal level of insulin production. This can greatly reduce a person's risk of diabetes and studies have shown that diabetes patients can even reduce the medication they take on a keto diet! When the body has a high carbohydrates intake, blood sugar quickly rises then works in overtime to bring the level back down. When this happens, the body produces cortisol, commonly called the "stress hormone". Often people with high blood sugar levels can have high amounts of this hormone which can cause things like dizziness, headaches, and irritability. With the keto diet, the body regulates the blood sugar and reduces the presence of cortisol. This takes the stress of your adrenal glands where the hormone is produced. The glands work to only produce the hormone when necessary instead of having to crank into action anytime there's a spike in your blood sugar. This results in the right hormones being produced at the right times.

When it comes to reproductive hormone issues, PCOS or Polycystic Ovary Syndrome is a condition that occurs in women and can lead to issues like disrupted menstrual cycles and infertility. It can be a heartbreaking diagnosis especially for couples who are trying to conceive. There is no cure for PCOS but the keto diet has become a popular method to try and correct this hormone imbalance. That's because PCOS is commonly associated with things like obesity, insulin resistance, and high blood glucose levels. Numerous studies have shown that women on a keto diet lifestyle have shown remarkable improvements in the areas of those symptoms. This can lead to regulating their insulin and hormone levels and an overall better quality of life. Regulating this hormone imbalance can increase a person's chance in having a successful pregnancy.

The keto diet has even been shown to have a positive effect on reducing the symptoms of PMS (pre-menstrual syndrome) that women can experience before their menstrual cycle. Acne, irritability, mood swings, headaches... these things can occur at times of hormone surges. Following a healthy ketogenic diet can regulate a woman's hormone levels at this time of the month.

Ketones are also a great way to regulate your immune system. They could be the key to healing other organs involved in diseases. For example, some diseases like hypothyroidism or autoimmune diseases occur when the body's organs turn on itself. It's not the organ's fault, but the immune system incorrectly tells it to attack the organ as if it's an invader. Ketone production is a great way to heal your immune system which can eventually lead to curing your hormone balance and regaining control of your immune system.

The way that the keto diet regulates hormones is by being a diet of high-quality fats and proteins. Hormones are composed of lipids (the scientific term for fat molecules), amino acids (protein molecules), and cholesterol. Sex hormones, in particular, are created by cholesterol and saturated fat. The ketogenic involves eating a high-quality diet of all of the above nutrients! This perfectly correlates to the production of high-quality hormones.

Think of it this way — the keto diet is set up to allow your body to naturally form ketones to use as energy. This is the same action the body would take if there were no carbohydrates to consume — keto followers are just voluntarily making the decision. The human body is a marvel that has been perfected by evolution to adapt to changing circumstances. If there is a shortage of carbohydrates for producing glucose energy, the body will naturally fall into a state of ketosis to use ketones as energy instead. This process would occur naturally and the body's hormone levels would adapt to it. A keto diet just capitalizes on the knowledge of ketosis and guides the body in that direction by maintaining a healthy keto diet.

Chapter 2:

How to Follow the Keto Diet

Fats and Carbs on the Keto Diet

The keto diet's goal is to limit the amount of carbohydrates consumption and increase the intake of healthy fats to quench your hunger. Macronutrients are the body's energy building blocks of carbs, fats, and proteins. Every person has their individual ratio of macronutrients in a day. Most people get half their energy from carbohydrates alone! The "average" diet consists of roughly 50% carbohydrates, 30% protein, and 20% fats. This depends on how healthy an eater you are! What the keto diet does is change the ratio of these nutrients to about 75% fats, 20% protein, and ~5% carbohydrates. By limiting the amount of carbs, the macro intake is changed so that the intake of the other two groups alone can meet your daily calorie requirement. With low carbs, the body begins the natural state of ketosis and burns ketones from the fat molecules you already have stored away. That means you lose weight!

One of the key points of a keto diet is restricting your carb intake to less than 50 grams of net carbs a day. If you have 25 grams of carbs but 5 grams of that is fiber, then you have a total net carb of 20 grams. The list of carbohydrates includes many items like bread, beans, pasta, rice, and sugar. You're surrounded by them! When first embarking on a keto diet, you'll feel the loss of carbohydrates instantly and painfully! What you want to do is incorporate more protein into your diet and fill up your day with healthy snacks like nuts and yogurt.

Recommended fats to eat include olive oil, coconut oil, and grass-fed butter products. You want to avoid trans fats which are harmful to the body and are proven to increase LDL or "bad" cholesterol levels. Mono-saturated and saturated fats are proven to be healthier. That includes meat and dairy products and things like nuts, almonds, avocados, olives, and eggs. Omega 3 fatty acids are also known to have a variety of health benefits. Fish, seafood walnuts, chia, and sunflower seeds are a great source of fatty acids.

Fats will comprise most of your diet on a keto plan so you want to make your meal choices with your favorite snacks in mind. You can add fat to your meals in the form of a salad dressing mixed with olive oil or adding a slice of organic butter on top of your meat. You can add fats even during the cooking process by being sure to use healthy fats like coconut oil, avocado oil, or ghee.

Ready for Keto?

If you're serious about starting a keto diet, you have to make a firm decision how intensely you will start your diet and then begin to clean out your pantry! Chances are carbs are everywhere! You want to first plan how fast you want to achieve entering the state of ketosis which will depend on how quickly you drastically reduce carbs in your diet. The more restrictive you are like having less than 15 grams a day, the faster your body will enter into a state of ketosis and begin producing ketones for energy. If you're still nervous about starting the diet and immediately cutting your carbs ratio, work your way down over a few days as you become comfortable with your new plans. It's up to you how you want to approach it!

When it comes to the actual meals, you will need to have a fridge and pantry stocked with keto-friendly ingredients. Planning your meals in advance is a great way to avoid the temptation of fast food or eating something not keto-friendly (like if other food is available at home if you don't live alone). By keeping a list of keto friendly ingredients at home, you can quickly whip up a keto dish at meal times. First, you need to get rid of what you don't need. You should not have grains, wheat or foods high in starch around. Things like bread, pasta, cereal, beans, potatoes.... you might consider them ordinary, but they're all high in refined carbohydrates which you need to cut out on your diet!

Don't forget the sugars! Not just the candies and sweet treats but also things like honey, maple syrup, or agave syrup. Sweetener substitutes can be used instead of granulated sugar. They're a great way to fool your body with a little sweet treat without taking in any sugars.

Now that you've gotten rid of temptations and you know exactly what you don't need to have around, it's time to go grocery shopping and get what you need! Researching some keto-friendly recipes is a great way to get an idea of what kind of meals you can eat and what new ingredients you might need to shop for. Whether it's buying organic, grass-fed meats, or switching to healthier oils like avocado or coconut, it's time to make a list and fill your pantries with keto-friendly items!

A Balanced Keto Diet

More often than not, when we think of dieting, you think of depriving yourself or going hungry with smaller portion sizes. There are so many diets that say no desserts or no protein! And yes, the keto diet does drastically reduce your carbohydrates intake, but it encourages a variety of healthy foods from different food groups that you can eat. When you see the list of keto-friendly items, you'll see just how many items you are still "allowed" to eat and can get creative about incorporating them into your meals.

The keto diet urges you to concentrate on consuming high energy foods and foods that are rich in fat such as meats, nuts, dairy, and vegetables. Fish, beef, eggs, and poultry are a great way to gain lots of protein and all the healthy fats that these foods offer. Vegetables also contain lots of amino acids and healthy minerals and vitamins that your body cannot do without. When it comes to snack time, the keto diet provides you with lots of alternatives to processed or junk foods that you may have relied on before. Healthy foods like nuts and cheeses are encouraged as snacks. Walnuts, pistachios, almonds... all these are great sources of healthy fats that can increase your "good cholesterol" number. Yogurt is rich with probiotics that keep your gut and digestive tract healthy. It's all about having a balanced diet that you enjoy but still fits with your macronutrient requirements.

Here are some examples!

Protein: You can keep the regular protein items that you would eat during your meals for your keto diet. If you're a meat lover — that's great! Fish is your favorite? It's considered even better for your health! In fact, meat, beef, seafood, and poultry are all great sources of energy and are perfect for the protein slot of your keto macro counts. Fish is also a rich source of amino acids and omega 3 fatty acids. Eggs are also a great snack that is rich in protein and hard-boiled eggs can be prepared in a matter of minutes. Try and buy organic grass-fed meat as much as you can so that you are minimizing any possible hormone or steroid intake through the food. But be warned — you don't want to have too much protein either on a keto diet, otherwise, that can slow your ketone production. Keeping track of your macros is extremely necessary so you know exactly how much protein you are taking in.

- Beef: steak, veal, ground beef
- Poultry: turkey, chicken, quail, duck
- Fish: mackerel, tuna, salmon, cod, catfish, halibut
- Shellfish: oysters, clams, crab, mussels, lobster
- Organ meats: liver, tongue, kidney, heart
- Pork: tenderloin, chops, ham, bacon, ground pork
- Lamb meat
- Goat meat

Vegetables and fruits grown underground tend to have a higher carb count so it's important to monitor those when you're on your keto diet. Once you have the hang of it, you'll easily be able to remember which are encouraged and which aren't! The other vegetables and fruits can still be eaten in moderation, though you want to avoid starchy vegetables that are high in carbs (yams, potatoes, corns, peas, beans, legumes, sweet potatoes). It's all about knowing how much you're eating and being careful to count your carbs so you are not taking in too many.

Vegetables: Broccoli, spinach, lettuce, bell pepper, celery, arugula, cauliflower, mushrooms... all are allowed! Leafy, dark green vegetables are especially great for keto-friendly meals and to make a generous salad topped with your favorite olive oil dressing. All these vegetables are high in nutrients but low in carbohydrates so they fit the keto profile. Zucchini, lettuce, and cucumbers are also great additions to your favorite healthy salads! The quickest meal is to toss together a quick salad of your favorite vegetables, maybe even adding some protein like chicken or ground beef. But sautéing or grilling veggies as a side with protein is a great way to have them too!

1 cup	*carbs*
Snow Peas	4.95 grams
Green Beans	4.27 grams
Cabbage	3 grams
Cauliflower	2.97 grams
Broccoli	4.04 grams
Brussel Sprouts	Sprouts 5.15 grams
Kale	5.15 grams
Zucchini	2.11 grams
Arugula	2.05 grams
Mushrooms	2.26 grams
Asparagus	1.78 grams
Spinach	1.43 grams
Celery	1.37 grams
Bok Choy	1.18 grams
Broccoli Rabe	Rabe 0.15 grams
Eggplant	2.88 grams
Bell Pepper	2.9 grams
Okra	4.25 grams
Bamboo Shoots	3 grams
Pumpkin	6 grams
Carrots	6.78 grams
Onion	7.64 grams

Fruits: Finding keto-friendly fruits can be a little trickier since fruits do tend to be high in carbohydrates. Especially when it comes to keeping track of net carbs, it can seem like a handful of fruits like a cup of blueberries can fill up your daily carb intake! But there are fruits that fit the keto profile and you can incorporate them into your diet. Avocados are one of the most heart-healthy fruits with tons of health benefits. Berries like raspberries, strawberries, and blackberries are a source of natural sugar but they are lower in carbs. Lemon is also fine. Not to say you'll be sucking on a lemon wedge, but fresh lemon juice squeezed over a salad or infused into water is a great idea! Tomatoes also are low in carbohydrates with only about 2 grams of net carbs in half a cup. They are great to incorporate into salads or as a side! Also, olives aren't necessarily the first thing you think of when you think of "fruit", but they are a fruit and are packed with fat and low in carbs — perfect for keto!

1 cup	*carbs*
Grapes	26 grams
Oranges	12 grams
Kiwi	9 grams
Strawberries	8 grams
Lemon	6 grams
Blueberries	17 grams
Pineapple	20 grams
Pear	22 grams
Banana	24 grams

Dairy: Dairy products play an important role in the keto diet. Try and find organic dairy products and ones with "full-fat" instead of the fat-free or low-fat options. That way, you are having a higher fat intake to fulfill your keto macros. Greek yogurt and soft cheeses like mozzarella and Colby can make a great snack with deli meats, while hard cheeses like parmesan, cheddar, and feta are great to add on salads. Cottage cheese, cream cheese, and mayo are also great for spreads. Butter and ghee are great alternatives too with about identical macronutrient contents — leaving it purely up to your preference! Ghee is a butter that has been clarified and tends to have a toastier, nutty flavor. Dairy also contains protein so you want to be sure of your protein intake when you pair it with a meal or a side. Evaporated and condensed milk should be avoided as they have high sugar contents!

1 cup	Carbs
Half-n-half	25 grams fat 7.6 grams protein 11.4 grams carbs
Greek yogurt	8 grams fat 22 grams protein 8 grams sugar
Sour cream	44 grams fat 5 grams protein 8 grams sugar
Mozzarella	0.6 grams carbs
Butter	184 grams fat 2 grams protein 0.1 grams sugar
Ghee	184 grams fat 2 grams protein 0.1 grams sugar
Full-fat cottage cheese	4 grams fat 3 grams carbs

Beverages: Water will be your main source of hydration on a keto diet but you can also enjoy coffee and tea. Almond or coconut milk is a great staple to include in your diet, especially if you are going to be making smoothies. They are a great unsweetened base. There are even some alcohols that you can have though you want to be sure you are ensuring moderation. Just be sure to avoid using sugar in your beverages and avoid anything like sweetened water. You can use substitute sugar sweeteners if you can't handle your morning coffee without sugar! Infusing your water with keto-friendly fruits like berries or lemons is a great alternative to skip the sugar but have some naturally sweetened water.

1 cup	*carbs*
Club soda 1 can	0 grams
Caffeinated tea	0 grams
Decaffeinated tea	0 grams
Lemon juice	3.31 grams
Lime juice	3.31 grams
Unsweetened almond milk	1.52 grams
Unsweetened hemp milk	1 gram

	carbs
Beer (light) 12 oz	3 grams
Bourbon 1 oz	0.03 grams
Gin 1 oz.	0 grams
Rum 1 oz.	0 grams
Scotch 1 oz	0 grams
Vodka 1 oz	0 grams
Wine (red) 5 oz	3.84 grams
Wine (white) 5 oz	3.83 grams
Champagne 3.5 oz	2.9 grams

Dessert: You can have chocolate on a keto diet! You want to stick to dark chocolates with about 70% raw cacaos or higher. So, if you are craving for sugar, this is a great way to have your "fix" and still remain on your diet!

Chapter 3:

Keto Meal Plans

Meal Plans

If you're ready to start the keto diet, you need to have a plan to work with! After cleaning out your pantry and going shopping for keto-friendly ingredients, it's time to plan your meals and snacks. People who feel they don't know what to eat or how to prepare a keto-friendly meal can be tempted to break the diet and have a meal loaded with high carbs instead.

One of the reasons people love the keto plan is because tracking your calories every day isn't required. Filling up on healthy fats and proteins means that your hunger is quenched and you're feeling full for longer. But as a beginner, it's a great idea to keep track of your meals and snacks so that you are not breaking the keto macro count. You want to stick at about 75% fat, 20% protein, ~5% carbohydrates, though some say 70/20/10 ratio works just as well. You want to be sure you're sticking consistently with that ratio daily in order for your body to recognize the cut in carbs and start the process of ketosis. You want to be sure you're not overeating on carbs, but also be sure you're eating enough protein and fats. If you're eating enough high-quality fats, you shouldn't feel hungry and can fight through the symptoms of the keto flu as your body adjusts.

How often you eat throughout the day depends on you. A keto diet has tons of recipes you can make for breakfast, lunch, and dinner so most people continue to have all three meals with light snacking in between. This ensures that you're getting your mix of protein and fat throughout the day to stay sated. But the best thing is to listen to your body! If you need to break up your meals to 5 to 6 small portions a day or if you're fine with a big breakfast and dinner, that works too. If you are physically active to lose weight faster, then you might need to spread out your meals to ensure you are eating enough after working out.

Here are some sample recipes to get you started!

BREAKFAST

Avocado and Egg Fat Bombs (2 servings, 2.5 grams carbs, 1.2 grams fiber, 1.2 grams protein, 15 grams fat, 1.3 grams net carbs)

.25 cup mayonnaise
a pinch of salt
a pinch of black pepper
1 teaspoon lemon or lime juice
half of an avocado, peeled and diced
3 egg yolks, cooked

Hard boil your eggs in water for about 10 minutes or using your electric egg boiler. You want only the yolk portion so remove that to use for this recipe. In a food processor, add your avocado, lemon or lime juice, mayonnaise, salt and pepper seasonings, and the three egg yolks. Pulse the food processor until the mixture is smooth. You can spoon this back into your egg white halves to make a keto friendly deviled egg.

Spinach and Cheese Omelet (2 servings: 510 calories, 42 grams fat, 30 grams protein, 11 grams net carbs)

3 large eggs
1 tablespoon feta cheese
.25 cup half and half milk
1 cup spinach leaves
2 sausages, cubed
.5 teaspoon olive oil
a pinch of salt
a pinch of black pepper

Scramble your eggs in a bowl with salt, pepper, and a half and half milk. In a skillet on a medium pan, add the olive oil to the pan. Add your sausage to the pan and let it brown. Add your spinach in next and sauté with some salt. Once both meat and spinach are cooked, take it out of the pan and add your egg mixture. When it looks like the omelet is cooking and turning light brown, add back in your spinach and meat. When the bottom side is done, flip the omelet and let the other side cook.

Bacon and Eggs (2 servings total, 1 serving: 270 calories, 3 grams carbs, 0 grams fiber, 22 grams fat, 19 grams protein)

4 eggs
3 ounces bacon, in slices
.25 cup sliced tomatoes

In a pan on medium heat, fry your bacon until it is crispy. Remove from heat once done. You can use the same pan to cook your eggs how you prefer them (cooked over easy, scrambled, sunny side up). Add in your tomatoes and fry them lightly. Add salt and pepper to your taste on top.

Mushroom Omelet (1 serving total, 510 calories, 40 grams fat, 28 grams protein, 6 grams carbs, 2 grams fiber, 4 grams net carbs)

1 ounce butter for frying the egg
1 ounce shredded cheese, Mozzarella or Cheddar
3 tablespoons chopped white onion
3 mushrooms, chopped
3 eggs
salt and pepper to your taste

Crack your eggs and mix with salt and pepper seasoning. In a skillet on low heat, melt the butter and add your egg mixture. When the egg begins to cook, add the cheese, mushrooms, and onion. Flip the omelet when the bottom has turned golden brown and cook the other side.

Coconut Porridge (1 serving total, 400 calories, 49 grams fat, 9 grams protein, 9 grams carbs, 5 grams fiber, 4 grams net carbs)

1 tablespoon coconut flour
1 tablespoon coconut oil
a pinch of husk powder
4 tablespoons coconut cream
a pinch of salt
1 egg

Add all your ingredients to a non-stick pan on low heat. Mix well until combined and continue stirring until you achieve a porridge-like texture. You can add some berries like strawberries or blueberries on top!

Avocado and Lime Smoothie (1 serving total, 30 grams fat, 15 grams carbs, 5 grams fiber, 28 grams protein, 10 grams net carbs)

1 lime juiced
.25 cup water
1 cup Greek yogurt
half an avocado pitted and peeled
1 tablespoon olive oil
2 tablespoons basil

Mix all ingredients in a blender until smooth!

Coconut Pancakes (2 servings, 578 calories, 50 grams fat, 20 grams protein, 3.5 grams net carbs)

2 eggs
.5 tablespoon erythritol or other sweetener substitutes
2 ounces cream cheese

a pinch of cinnamon
1 tablespoon almond flour
a pinch of salt

Crack and whisk your eggs in a large mixing bowl. Add the cream cheese in first so it is well mixed then add the erythritol, salt, almond flour, and cinnamon. In a skillet on medium heat, add about half the pancake batter and let it cook until the edges begin to brown slightly. This can be about 3-4 minutes so ensure you are watching patiently to avoid burning the pancake. Flip carefully and brown the other side then remove from heat. Do this with the other half of the batter. You can add berries or coconut flakes as a topping.

Keto Blueberry Muffins (12 servings total, 247 calories per serving, 21.8 grams fat, 7.3 grams protein, 9.3 grams carbs, 2.9 grams fiber, 5.4 grams net carbs)

1 teaspoon sea salt
1 teaspoon baking soda
1 tablespoon baking powder
.75 cup artificial keto-friendly sweetener of your choice
7 tablespoons coconut oil
3 large eggs at room temperature
1.5 teaspoons vanilla extract
.75 cup fresh blueberries
3 cups almond flour
4 tablespoons coconut flour
.5 cup unsweetened applesauce

Preheat your oven to 350 degrees F and spray a muffin tin with cooking spray or line with liners. Mix together your dry ingredients in a bowl — baking soda, salt, baking powder, coconut, and almond flour. Mix your dry ingredients with a hand mixer until smooth — the sweetener, coconut oil, eggs, applesauce, and vanilla extract. Stir in the almond flour into the wet ingredients and toss the blueberries in and stir gently. Let the batter rest for 10 minutes. Use a spoon or cookie scoop to divide the mixture into the muffin tray wells. Bake for about 25 minutes until the tops are golden brown.

Breakfast BLT Salad (2 servings total, 292 calories per serving, 18 grams carbohydrates, 7 grams fiber, 17.5 grams protein, 18 grams fat)

2 eggs
4 strips cooked bacon, crumbled
a quarter of an avocado, sliced
10 grape tomatoes
salt and pepper to taste
3 cups shredded kale
2 teaspoons extra virgin olive oil
1 teaspoon vinegar

Combine the kale, olive oil, and salt and pepper in a bowl. Stir well until the kale softens. Cook your eggs however you like — boiled works great for this recipe but scrambled is also good! Add the bacon, tomatoes, avocado, and egg on top of the kale.

Avocado Smoothie with Ginger and Turmeric (2 servings total, 208 calories per serving, 21 grams fat, 5 grams carbs, 1 gram fiber, 4 grams net carbs)

half an avocado pitted and peeled
.5 teaspoon turmeric
1 teaspoon lemon or lime juice
1 cup crushed ice
1-2 teaspoons keto-friendly sweetener to your taste
1 teaspoon freshly minced ginger

.25 cup almond mink
.75 cup full fat coconut milk

Add all your ingredients except the ice and sweetener in the blender and blend until smooth. Once the ingredients are well mixed, add the crushed ice and sweetener. Blend until all ingredients are combined!

LUNCH

Turkey Chili with Cauliflower Rice Bowl (4 servings total, 2 servings: 390 calories, 30 grams protein, 34 grams fat, 7 grams carbohydrates)

1 pound organic ground turkey
2 cups coconut milk
2 cups cauliflower rice
1 teaspoon of salt, thyme, garlic powder, black pepper, paprika
2 garlic cloves
1 cup diced onion
3 tablespoons coconut oil

Heat your coconut oil in a large pot. Add your garlic and onion when the oil is hot and you smell the aroma of the garlic. Add your turkey and spices and stir until well combined. Next, add the cauliflower rice. Stir the mixture until the turkey is golden brown. Then add your coconut milk and bring the mixture to a boil. Keep stirring to avoid burning. Reduce the heat for 10-15 minutes then remove from heat.

Deli Meat Plate (2 servings total, 1 serving: 822 calories, 40 grams protein, 59 grams fat, 3 grams fiber, 11 grams carbs, 8 grams net carbs)

10 green or black olives
7 ounces prosciutto, sliced
7 ounces mozzarella cheese
salt and pepper to taste
.25 cup olive oil
2 tomatoes sliced

Arrange the tomatoes, cheese, olives, and prosciutto in a platter. Sprinkle with salt and pepper and olive oil.

Mushroom Bacon Skillet (2 servings total, 213 calories per serving, 8.5 grams fat, 13.6 grams protein, 8.4 grams carbs, 0.3 grams fiber, 8.1 grams net carbs)

.5 teaspoon dried thyme
1 tablespoon minced garlic
.5 teaspoon salt
2 cups halved mushrooms (shiitake, cremini, and ali'i mushrooms are a great combination)
4-5 slices bacon

Prepare your ingredients by cutting the bacon into half inch pieces and slicing the mushrooms in half. Heat a large skillet over medium heat. Once the pan has heated, add the bacon to the skillet and cook until it is crispy. Move to the side and add the mushrooms in and sauté until golden brown. Once the mushrooms soften, add your seasoning - salt, thyme, garlic. Keep stirring for another 5-7 minutes until everything is well combined. Remove from heat.

Keto Friendly Pizza Rolls (3 servings total, 117 calories, 3 grams carbs, 8 grams fat, 10 grams protein, 1 gram fiber, 2 grams net carbs)

.25 cup chopped bell peppers
1 tablespoon white onion, diced
.25 cup meat topping of your choice whether crumbled sausage or pepperoni
.5 teaspoon pizza seasoning
1 cup mozzarella cheese
.5 cup pizza sauce, one low in carbs
.25 cup tomatoes, sliced

Line your baking sheet with parchment paper and set your oven to 400 degrees F. You can use just a few drops of olive oil on the parchment paper so your dish does not stick. First, sprinkle out your cheese all over the pan in a single layer. Make sure there aren't any holes or gaps in the layer. Then add the pizza seasoning. Bake in the oven for about 15 minutes or until the cheese is golden brown. Remove from the oven and add your toppings of tomato slices, onions, bell pepper, and meat of choice. Drizzle the tomato sauce on top. Place back in the oven for another 12-15 minutes or until the top is golden brown and how you prefer your pizza.

Bacon, Avocado, Cheese Salad (2 servings total, 1 serving: 890 calories, 89 grams fat, 15 grams carbs, 27 grams protein, 9 grams fiber, 6 grams total net carbs)

1 avocado peeled and diced
.5 cup bacon, cooked and crumbled
.5 cup goat cheese
.25 cup chopped walnuts, unsalted
.5 cup lettuce

Preheat your oven to 400 degrees F. Line a baking sheet with parchment paper. Slice your goat cheese into pieces and bake for about 2-3 minutes until light brown. If you haven't already, you can brown your bacon in the oven too or in a skillet on medium heat if you prefer. Toss together the lettuce and avocado and add your bacon and cheese on top. Top with walnuts. For dressing, use 2 tablespoons of olive oil with equal amounts of vinegar and a squirt of lemon juice. Add salt and pepper to your taste.

Chocolate Almond Smoothie (1 serving total, 178 calories, 12.8 grams total fat, 6.8 grams carbs, 10.1 grams protein, 2.4 grams fiber, 4.4 total net carbs)

3 drops Stevia liquid
1 tablespoon cocoa powder, unsweetened
1 cup almond milk
.75 cup water
1.5 tablespoon almond butter
.25 cup cottage cheese

Blend all the ingredients in a blender until smooth!

Keto Friendly Fruit Salad

1 cup fresh blueberries
1 cup fresh strawberries
.5 cup feta cheese, crumbled
salt and pepper to taste
1 small bunch of kale leaves
2 tablespoons olive oil
2 tablespoons lemon or lime juice

If you prefer to remove the tough stems from the kale, you can do so at this time. Chop the leaves up finely. In a large salad bowl, combine the kale with olive oil and salt and mix thoroughly until the kale softens. Add the lemon juice and black pepper. Add the strawberries, blueberries, and feta cheese. Mix until everything is well combined.

Pesto Chicken Salad (4 servings total, each serving: 375 calories, 29 grams fat, 22 grams protein, 3 grams net carbs)

1 pound chicken, cooked and cubed
1 avocado, peeled and diced
.25 cup tomato slices
2 tablespoons green pesto
8 slices bacon, cooked and crumbled into pieces
1 teaspoon olive oil
a pinch of salt
a pinch of black pepper
Combine all ingredients in a mixing bowl. Toss with the olive oil and the salt and pepper seasoning.

Tuna Salad and Boiled Eggs (2 servings total, 1 serving:900 calories, 30 grams protein, 90 grams fat, 10 grams carbs, 5 grams protein, 5 grams net carbs)

4 eggs
.5 pound lettuce
4 ounces celery
6 ounces tuna
1 cup cherry tomatoes
2 tablespoons olive oil
salt and pepper to taste
2 tablespoons lemon juice
.75 cup mayonnaise

Rinse and then dice your celery sticks and add to a bowl of the tuna, lemon juice, and mayonnaise. Add salt and pepper to your taste. Boil your eggs for about 7-9 minutes until hardboiled. Peel and halve. Place your tuna mixture and eggs on top of your shredded lettuce. Add the cherry tomatoes and drizzle with olive oil. Add additional salt and pepper if you'd like or a pinch of paprika can provide a taste of heat!

DINNER

Mushroom Chicken (2 servings total, 1 serving: 330 calories, 21 grams protein, 28 grams fat, 4 grams carbs)

2 chicken breast cuts
1 small onion
5 large mushrooms
.5 teaspoon Himalayan salt
.25 cup coconut milk
2 tablespoons butter
salt and pepper to taste
1 teaspoon dried herbs

Slice your vegetables while you have a skillet warming up on medium heat. Once it is hot, add in half of the butter and let it melt. Once it's melted, add the vegetables and season them with salt and pepper. Stir until the vegetables become soft then remove from the heat. Add the rest of the butter and let it melt. While you wait, season your chicken with the Himalayan salt and the dried herbs. Cook the chicken in the skillet for about 5-7 minutes or as you prefer. Add the veggie mixture back into the pan and top the dish with coconut milk. Let the pan simmer for a few minutes until everything is well combined. Remove from heat.

Shrimp Stir Fry with Baked Cauliflower Rice (4 servings total, 357 calories per serving, 24.8 grams fat, 9 grams carbs, 24.7 grams protein)

2 tablespoons MCT oil
12 oz frozen cauliflower rice
4 stalks green onions
5-6 mushrooms

3 garlic cloves
3 tablespoons bacon fat (or butter, ghee)
1-inch lemon rind
2-inch ginger root
1 pound shrimp, peeled, tail on
2 teaspoons Himalayan pink salt

Preheat your oven to 400 degrees F to roast the cauliflower rice. Spread the rice on a sheet pan and drizzle with the MCT oil. Sprinkle the pink salt to your flavoring. Bake for 10 minutes in the oven. Slice your ginger and garlic into small pieces and slice your green onion too. In a large skillet, add the bacon fat on medium heat. Add your ginger, garlic, and green onion and stir until fragrant and soft. Add the shrimp and sauté until they are pink. Add the salt and stir another few minutes. Remove from heat. Serve with the cauliflower rice. Garnish with more green onions or veggies as you prefer.

Steak Stir Fry (4 servings total, 290 calories per serving, 11 grams fat, 38.5 grams protein, 6 grams net carbs)

2 cloves minced garlic
1 small onion sliced
1 small bell pepper sliced
.25 cup mushrooms sliced
1 cup beef broth
1 teaspoon grated ginger
1 tablespoon olive oil
1 pound beef sirloin
2 tablespoons low carb soy sauce
salt and pepper

First, add the olive oil to a large skillet over medium heat. Once the oil heats up, add the beef and crumble in the pan. Add ginger and garlic to season. Let it brown for about 5 minutes. Season with salt and pepper. Remove from heat and add the peppers and onions. Stir the vegetables for about 3-5 minutes until they become soft. Add in the mushrooms and stir until they are soft. Add the beef broth and soy sauce and return the beef to the cook. Let simmer for a few minutes then remove from heat.

Baked Cilantro Meatballs

1 egg
.3 cup coconut flour
1 pound ground beef
3 spring onions, finely chopped
12-15 pieces of cilantro, finely chopped
salt and pepper to taste
3 tablespoons olive oil

Preheat your oven to 440 degrees F. Mix the ground beef with the cilantro, spring onions, salt, and pepper. Lightly oil your fingers so you can handle the meat as you form regular sized meatballs. Use a spoon to equally portion them out. Lightly dip the meatballs in the coconut flour and arrange on a baking sheet lined with parchment paper. Bake for about 10-15 minutes in the oven until golden brown. Serve with a side of veggies or crumble over a Caesar salad.

Low Carb Meat Loaf (6 servings total, 2 servings: 344 calories, 32 grams fat, 31 grams protein, 6 grams carbs, 2 grams fiber, 4 total net carbs)

2 eggs
1 tablespoon lemon zest
.25 cup chopped parsley
2 pounds 85% grass-fed ground beef

.25 cup chopped basil
1 teaspoon salt
1 teaspoon black pepper
3-4 cloves garlic
2 tablespoons avocado oil

Set your oven to 400 degrees F. In a large bowl, combine your beef with the salt and pepper seasoning. In a blender, combine your eggs, herbs, garlic, and the oil. Blend until the eggs are frothy and the garlic and herbs are well combined. Add the egg to your beef and mix until well incorporated. Transfer the meat to a small 8x4 or 9x5 baking pan. Smooth the edges and flatten with a spatula or your hands. Bake for 50-65 minutes depending on how lightly golden brown the top has become.

Crispy Chicken Thighs (6 servings total, 1 serving: 404 calories, 35 grams fat, 0.8 total carbs, 22.8 grams protein, 0.1 grams fiber, 0.7 grams net carbs)

1 cup butter
1 teaspoon cream of tartar
6 ~4 oz chicken thighs with the skin on
1 tablespoon paprika
.5 teaspoon baking soda
salt and pepper to taste
Heat your oven to 400 degrees F. You want to dry your chicken legs so pat out the moisture with a towel or paper towels. Arrange the legs on a baking sheet or 2 sheets if your sheet is too small. Underneath the skin, add butter and add butter on top of the chicken too. Combine your spices and cream of tartar in a bowl. Add salt and pepper to your taste. Rub the mixture all over the chicken and bake for 25-35 minutes until the chicken skin is golden brown.

Creamy Mushroom Chicken (2 servings total, 334 calories per serving, 27.3 grams fat, 24.3 grams protein, 3.2 grams carbs)

6-7 mushrooms
1 small onion
.5 teaspoon dried thyme (or basil, oregano, herb you prefer)
.5 teaspoon Himalayan salt
2 tablespoons butter
.3 cup full fat coconut milk
2 chicken cutlets

Heat the butter in a skillet on medium heat while you dice your onion and mushrooms. Once the butter is melted, add in the sliced mushrooms and sprinkle with some salt. Sauté until brown and then add the onions. Keep stirring until soft. Remove the vegetable mix from the skillet. Add the last of the butter and let it melt. Sprinkle your chicken cutlets with the dried herb and salt. Place in the skillet and cook for 5-7 minutes on each side. Add the onion and mushroom mixture back into the skillet and pour the coconut milk on top. Let it simmer for a few minutes then remove from heat.

Low Carb Keto Lasagna (6 servings total, 364 calories per serving, 21 grams fat, 12 grams carbs, 32 grams protein)

15 oz ricotta cheese
.5 pound Italian sausage
1 egg
salt and pepper to taste
1 teaspoon garlic powder
2 tablespoons coconut flour
1 tablespoon butter or ghee (coconut oil or lard can also be used)
1 clove of garlic

1.25 cup mozzarella cheese
.25 cup parmesan cheese
4 large zucchinis sliced horizontally
16 oz low carb marinara sauce
2 tablespoon mixed Italian herb seasonings

Preheat your oven to 375 degrees F and coat a 9x9 baking dish with butter. First, you want to treat your zucchini to some salt seasoning for flavor. Heat the 1 tablespoon of butter (or whichever fat you chose) in a large skillet. Add in the sausage once the oil is hot and cook until golden brown. Remove from heat and let it cool as you prepare your lasagna base. Mix the ricotta cheese, egg, 1 cup of mozzarella cheese, 2 tablespoons of parmesan cheese, coconut flour, garlic, garlic powder, salt, and pepper until mixed. Add the Italian seasoning. Arrange your sliced zucchini at the bottom of the dish and spread about .25 cup of the cheese mixture, then add .25 cup of the Italian sausage, then add the marinara sauce. Continue this layering until you've used up all the ingredients — you should have about 3-4 layers. Add the remaining mozzarella and parmesan cheese on top. Cover with aluminum foil and bake for 30 minutes. Remove the foil then bake for an additional 15 minutes until the top is golden brown.

Baked Salmon Steaks (2 servings total, 1 serving: 420 calories, 3.4 grams carbs, 21 grams protein, 37 grams fat, 0.1 grams fiber, 3.3 grams net carbs)

salt to taste
black pepper to taste
3 tablespoons lemon juice
.25 cup melted better
2 salmon steaks
1 tablespoon Worcestershire sauce

First, you want to marinate your salmon in the sauce you will create of the butter, Worcestershire sauce, salt and pepper to your taste, and the lemon juice. A great way to marinate is to prepare it in a ziplock bag and then add the salmon until it's soaked in the sauce. Let it soak for about 20-30 minutes. Then, preheat your oven to 400 degrees F. Lay your salmon steaks on a baking sheet lined with parchment paper. Bake for about 7-10 minutes. Remove from heat and drizzle the remainder of the marinade you made on top for seasoning. Allow it to bake for another 10 to 15 minutes until the fish becomes golden brown.

Pork Tenderloin with Spinach Side (6 servings total, 1 serving: 490 calories, 1.9 grams carbs, 42 grams fat, 0.7 grams fiber, 1.2 grams net carbs, 30 grams protein)

1 teaspoon avocado oil
salt and pepper to taste
1 cup spinach leaves
2-3 cloves of garlic
4 ounces cream cheese
1 pound pork tenderloin
1 teaspoon thyme
1 teaspoon paprika
5 ounces Gruyere cheese

Preheat your oven to 375 degrees F. Heat your avocado oil in a skillet and add the garlic cloves. Sauté until light brown and you smell the aroma of the garlic. Add spinach and sauté it until just wilted. Stir in the cream cheese and season with salt and pepper to your taste. Remove from the heat. Cut your pork tenderloin in half but not completely — you want to leave about half an inch remaining between the two sides. Cover with aluminum foil and pound the meat using a meat hammer. Add the meat tenderizer, thyme, paprika, Gruyere cheese, and other keto-friendly seasonings if you prefer (like cinnamon or garlic powder). Place your meat on a baking sheet and bake for about 40-50 minutes. Serve with the spinach as a side.

Chipotle Steak Bowl (4 servings total, 1 serving: 620 calories, 45 grams fat, 30 grams protein, 5.9 grams net carbs)

8-ounce high-quality grass-fed skirt steak
.5 cup sour cream
.25 cup pepper jack cheese or cheddar if you prefer
.5 cup guacamole
.5 teaspoon Tabasco sauce
salt and pepper to taste

Have a cast iron skillet on medium heat. Season your steak with salt and pepper as you prefer your meat seasoning. Cook on each side for about 5-7 minutes or to your liking. Remove from heat and once cool, cut into 4-5 pieces with a sharp steak knife. In a bowl, mix the shredded cheese, sour cream, tobacco sauce, and guacamole. Add the steak pieces on top.

Steak Dinner with Mushroom Sides (4 servings total, 1 serving: 508 calories, 7.02 grams carbs, 2.3 grams fiber, 38.07 grams protein, 4.7 total net carbs)

1.5 pounds high-quality grass-fed steaks
salt and pepper to taste
2-3 garlic cloves minced
.25 cup melted butter or ghee
8 ounces green beans
8 ounces mushrooms

You want to preheat your oven while you prep your vegetables. Trim the edges of your green beans and cut them into half. You can cut your mushrooms into halves if they are on the bigger side. Spread your veggies on a baking tray. Mix the butter or ghee with the minced garlic and drizzle half of that mixture over the veggies. Sprinkle with salt and pepper for further seasoning. Roast for about 12 minutes. Remove from heat once golden brown. Drizzle the rest of the butter mixture on the steaks. Rub in the seasoning. Broil the steaks in the same baking tray for about 5 minutes each side until they are done to your liking.

Need some more ideas? We have them for you!

Breakfast:
Omelet topped with mushroom, feta cheese, and spinach
Unsweetened yogurt with raspberries, walnuts, and chia seeds
Tomato, kale, bacon egg frittata
Scrambled eggs with avocado
Keto-friendly blueberry muffins
Classic bacon and scrambled eggs
Avocado and keto-friendly vegetable smoothie

Lunch:
Salad! All your favorite leafy green vegetables topped with cheese or meat of your choice. Avocado and boiled eggs are a great addition too.
Salmon with vegetable as a side like spinach or broccoli
Cauliflower crust pizza topped with keto-friendly vegetables and low-carb tomato sauce
Bacon & Cheese Soup
Lettuce wrap full of chicken, veggies, and nuts
Baked bell peppers stuffed with crab and cheese
Pesto chicken salad
Fruit salad of keto-friendly fruits like strawberries and blueberries

Dinner:
Chicken salad with strips of chicken breast
Grilled chicken with a vegetable side (squash, zucchini, spinach, tomatoes)
Ground beef meatloaf with low-carb tomato sauce
Bone Broth
Chicken and kale soup
Pan seared cod with a veggie side
Chicken pot pie casserole

Snacks:
Vegetables with cream cheese or nut butter dip
Keto chips
Devilled or hard-boiled eggs
Fat Bombs (see next section)
Flaxseed crackers
A handful of nuts like almonds, walnuts, or macadamia nuts
Chocolate mousse (heavy cream mixed with cocoa powder)
Beef jerky (make sure it's very low in carbs)
Avocado
Berries like strawberries, blueberries, or raspberries
Deli meat
Olives
Cheeses (string cheese, Colby cheese)
Pork rinds
Seeds (sunflower, chia, flax, pumpkin)
Dark chocolate w/ at least 80% cocoa content or higher
Seaweed snacks
Sardines
Pepperoni slices
Greek or full-fat yogurt

What are Fat Bombs?

If you've looked into the keto diet or had a friend or family follow the diet, you've probably heard the term "fat bomb". The term has become popular as the name given to a snack or meal replacement made out of keto-friendly ingredients meant to give dieters an instant pick me up! They can be sweet or savory! They contain a high fat content and are designed to fill you up and give you a boost of energy when you are following the keto diet plan. By being high in fat and low in protein, they drive the body towards ketosis to burn more fats for fuel.

If you are following a keto diet, you're sure to have the common ingredients to make fat bombs in your pantry already. They tend to be every day, inexpensive ingredients like nuts, eggs, butter, seeds, coconut flakes, cheese, and sour cream. You can even use keto-friendly dark chocolate for those sweet fat bombs! The most common ingredients that make up a fat bomb are usually coconut oil and high-fat dairy ingredients like ghee, butter, or cream cheese. The secret to a great fat bomb is softening your fat base like cheese or ghee and blending and mixing in the other ingredients to create a tasty, filling treat!

Coconut oil especially has been found to have many health benefits and provides the body with ketones. It is a fat that is absorbed quickly by the body and used as fuel for an instant boost of energy. Ingredients like cheese and butter contain other vitamins and minerals that are necessary for the body. Those high-quality dairy products have a fatty acid called CLA that has been found to prevent heart disease and decrease body fat. This fatty acid is found in higher quantities in dairy products that are made from 100% grass-fed cows. This is important to remember when shopping for your keto ingredients! Just like when choosing the best grass-fed and organic types of protein, you want to be sure you're using the highest quality dairy products for your fat bombs to ensure you have the highest fat content.

Fat bombs have become very popular in the keto diet because they allow you to eat something "unhealthy" that you might be craving (especially sweet treats!) while still sticking to your keto diet rules. That's considered a win-win! But you want to be sure you are sticking to your keto macro diet. Nearly 80% of your calories will come from fat. If you're already eating high-quality keto-friendly meals and snacking on high-fat snacks throughout the day, it's possible you've reached your caloric limit for fat. You might not even need keto bombs to hit your fat goal!

The key is to enjoy these treats in moderation. They are great as a snack or an appetizer or if you happen to have skipped a meal and need a quick pick-me-up. These are especially easy to have because recipes usually make nearly a dozen or so! They're easy to store and you can keep them refrigerated and get out when you have a craving. They will help you stay full longer because the high-fat content will quench your cravings. They will help you burn more fat for fuel and keep your body in a state of ketosis.

To help you on your keto diet journey, we have compiled some recipes for sweet and savory fat bombs — depending on which craving you might have! They are often prepared with simple keto-friendly ingredients and artificial sweeteners so you don't have to buy any special ingredients. You can create them in bulk. Most recipes often make 10-12 fat bombs and you can refrigerate or freeze them to eat as necessary.

SWEET FAT BOMBS

Keto Friendly Chocolate Fudge (10 servings total, 158 calories per serving, 13 grams fat, 4.2 grams carbs, 2.1 grams fiber, 2.1 grams net carbs)

Stevia or artificial sweetener sugar to your taste
1 teaspoon vanilla extract
.75 cup coconut butter
4 ounces 100% dark chocolate

Slowly melt the chocolate in the microwave or using the double broiler method. Melt the coconut butter the same way. In a medium size bowl, mix together the coconut butter, chocolate, and vanilla extract. Add sugar sweetener to your taste. Pour the mixture into a parchment lined baking sheet. Refrigerate for 1 hour or until the mixture has become solid. Remove from pan and cut into 10-12 pieces.

Coconut Chocolate Mounds Bars (4 servings total, 345 calories per serving, 18 grams fat, 5 grams protein, 7.2 grams carbs, 3.8 grams fiber, 3.4 grams net carbs)

.5 cup coconut oil
.5 cup organic coconut milk
.5 cup powdered sweetener
8 ounces 100% dark chocolate
1 cup unsweetened shredded coconut

Combine the coconut milk, coconut oil, and sweetener in a pan on low heat. Mix until well combined then add the coconut flakes. Line a baking sheet with parchment paper and spread the mixture into a tray. Refrigerate for 3 hours or until the mixture becomes solid. Gently hold the pan upside down press the bottom of the pan until the mixture comes out. Cut into 3" bars. Melt the chocolate using a microwave or double broiler method. Stir well and be sure there are no lumps. You will then dip your coconut bars into the melted chocolate. Let them rest on parchment paper until the chocolate hardens. Dipping the bars a second time is even better to add an extra chocolate layer. After the second dip, let them rest on parchment paper until the chocolate sets.

Cocoa and Cashew Fat Bombs (20 servings total, 133 calories per serving, 18 grams fat, 4 grams protein, 5.8 grams carbs, 1.1 grams fiber, 4.7 grams net carbs)

4 tablespoons coconut flour
.5 cup almond butter
.5 cup coconut oil
.5 cup cashews, unsalted
.25 cup unsweetened cocoa powder

Melt the coconut oil and almond butter in a skillet over low heat. Stir until evenly mixed. In a bowl, add the coconut and almond butter combination you just made and mix with the cocoa powder and coconut flour. Put the bowl in the freezer for about 15 minutes until the mixture cools. Use a food processor to ensure your cashews are in bite-size pieces. Take the mixture out of the freezer and form about half tablespoon size balls using a spoon or cookie scoop. Roll each ball in the cashews mixture until well coated. Refrigerate the fat bombs for 10-15 minutes or until they become hard.

Walnut and Orange Chocolate Fat Bombs (14 servings total, 87 calories per serving, 8.4 grams fat, 3 grams carbs, 1.5 grams protein, 1.5 grams net carbs, 1.42 grams fiber)

1 cup unsalted walnuts, chopped
1 tablespoon fresh orange zest or orange extract
4 ounces keto-friendly dark chocolate
.25 cup coconut oil
15-20 drops Stevia sugar sweetener to taste
a pinch of cinnamon powder

Microwave your chocolate or use a double boiler method to melt it. Stir consistently to make sure there are no lumps. Add the sugar, coconut oil, and cinnamon into the chocolate mixture. Add the sugar sweetener to your taste. Add the orange zest or orange extract, whichever you are using. Add the walnuts and mix until they are coated in the chocolate. Line a muffin tray with a paper cup or silicone liners. Spoon the mixture out evenly into 12-14 cups. Refrigerate the tray for 1 hour or until the mixture has solidified.

Vanilla Cheesecake Fat Bombs (14 servings total, 90 calories per serving, 10 grams fat, 1.9 grams fiber, 3.9 grams carbs, 2 grams net carbs)

1 brick (8-ounce package) of cream cheese, grass-fed
2 teaspoons vanilla extract
.5 cup Stevia sugar sweetener
1 cup heavy cream divided into 2 portions, grass-fed

Use a hand mixer to beat the vanilla extract, cream cheese, and sweetener together. Start on low speed for 2-3 minutes then increase the speed. Scrape the edges of the bowl so everything is well combined. Add half of the heavy cream to the mixture and beat until smooth. Set the bowl aside for 5 minutes so the sugar can dissolve. Add the last of the cream and mix until there are peaks forming at the top. It should take about 2-5 minutes more of mixing with the hand mixer. Line a muffin tray with paper cup liners or silicone liners. Use a cookie scoop to fill the liners evenly with the mixture. Place in the freezer for 1 hour or until mixture solidifies.

Chocolate Peanut Butter Cup Fat Bombs (10 servings total, 120 calories per serving, 9.8 grams fat, 5 grams total carbs, 3.2 grams fiber, 3.6 grams protein, 1.8 grams net carbs)

.25 teaspoon pink Himalayan salt
10 drops Stevia liquid sweetener
6 tablespoons creamy peanut butter
5 ounces keto-friendly dark chocolate

Line a muffin tray with paper or silicone liners. Melt your chocolate in the microwave. Be sure you're stirring consistently so there are no lumps! Add your peanut butter and liquid sweetener to the chocolate mixture and stir well to combine. Then pour into the liners and top with a few grains of the pink salt. Keep the tray refrigerated for 1 hour or until the mixture has solidified.

Peppermint Fat Bombs (14 servings total, 200 calories per serving, 22 grams fat, 2 grams carbs, 1.1 grams fiber, 0.9 grams net carbs)

2 tablespoons unsweetened cocoa
.5 cup and 2 tablespoons coconut oil, melted
2 tablespoons Stevia powdered sweetener
.25 cup peppermint extract

In a bowl, mix the peppermint extract and sweetener into the coconut oil. Mix until well combined. Pour half the mixture into a silicone mold try or in a muffin tray set with liners. This becomes the first layer of the snack. Place in the fridge for 15-

20 minutes until set. To the mixture, add the cocoa powder. Add the chocolate layer on top once the white layer has set. Place back in the fridge for 1 hour or until solidified.

Blueberry Fat Bombs (15 servings total, 52 calories per serving, 5.8 grams fat, 2.1 grams carbs, 0.8 grams fiber, 1.3 grams net carbs)

2.5 tablespoons Stevia sugar sweetener
3 ounces blueberries, fresh or frozen
1 cup cream cheese, grass-fed

You want to be sure your blueberries and cream cheese are soft at room temperature. In a blender, combine all the ingredients and blend until smooth. Keep refrigerated for 15-20 minutes until the mixture is more firm to roll into balls. Use a cookie scoop to make about 15 tablespoon size balls and place on a tray. Keep the tray refrigerated for 1 hour until frozen solid.

Macaroon Fat Bombs (12 servings total, 47 calories per serving, 5.1 grams fat, 3.0 grams carbs, 1.3 grams fiber, 1.7 grams net carbs)

.5 cup unsweetened shredded coconut
.3 cup organic almond flour
2 tablespoons Stevia sugar sweetener
2 teaspoons coconut oil, melted
2 teaspoons vanilla extract
3 egg whites

Set your oven to 400 degrees F. Keep an empty medium-sized bowl in the fridge to chill. This is what you will use to beat your eggs so they become frothy in a cool bowl. Until then, mix your coconut, Stevia sugar, and almond flour until well blended.

Add your coconut oil and vanilla extract to the mixture. Mix well. You can now whisk your egg whites in the chilled bowl. You want to whisk until the mixture forms stiff peaks. Gently fold the flour mixture into the egg whites. Try not to over mix! Use a cookie scoop to make about 10-12 portions and place on a parchment lined tray for baking. Bake for 10-12 minutes or until the macaroons lightly become brown at the top.

White Chocolate Fat Bombs (8 servings total, 125 calories per serving, 10 grams fat, 0 grams protein, 0 grams carbs)

10 drops Stevia sugar sweetener drops
.5 teaspoon vanilla extract
.25 cup coconut oil
.25 cup cocoa butter

Line a muffin tray with paper or silicone liners. Melt the cocoa butter and coconut oil in the microwave or using the double broiler method. Stir in the vanilla extract and the sugar sweetener drops. Pour the mixture into the liners and refrigerate for 1 hour or until mixture has solidified.

Raspberry and Nuts Chocolate Bark (8 servings total, 82 calories per serving, 7.3 grams fat, 3.2 grams carbs, 2 grams fiber, 1.2 grams net carbs)

.25 cup almond butter
1-2 teaspoons Stevia sugar powder
1 tablespoon unsweetened cocoa powder
.25 cup unsalted raw almonds
.5 cup coconut butter
.25 cup unsalted raw walnuts
.3 cup raspberries, fresh or frozen

Make sure your nuts are in small bite-size pieces. Mix together the sugar, cocoa powder, almond butter, and coconut butter in a bowl. Spread this mixture out into a parchment lined baking sheet. Use a spatula to spread it out evenly. Microwave the raspberries for about 30-50 seconds until the fruit becomes soft and releases some juices. Sprinkle the raspberries and chopped nuts over the chocolate. Keep the tray in the freezer for 1 hour or until the mixture hardens. Once frozen, use a sharp knife to cut into 8-10 pieces.

Gingerbread Fat Bombs (16 servings total, 120 calories per serving, 2.9 grams carbs, .9 grams fiber, 2 grams net carbs, 10.9 grams fat)

2 cups almond flour
a pinch of kosher salt
.5 teaspoon ground cinnamon powder
2/3 cup Stevia sugar sweetener
.25 teaspoon ground nutmeg powder
1 teaspoon ground ginger powder
.3 cup melted butter, grass-fed

Mix together all the dry ingredients (your spices and flour). Then, add the melted butter into the flour mixture and slowly mix until it forms a thick dough. Use a spoon to make about 16 balls and place onto a tray. Keep the tray refrigerated for 1 hour or until balls have solidified.

SAVORY FAT BOMBS

Savory Salmon Fat Bombs (6 servings total, 147 calories per serving, 15.9 grams fat, 1.0 grams carbs, 0.4 grams fiber, 0.6 grams net carbs)

.3 cup butter, grass-fed
2 ounces smoked salmon filet, about half a package
2 teaspoons lemon or lime juice
.5 cup cream cheese, grass-fed
2 tablespoons fresh dill or 1 tablespoon if using dried dill
a pinch of kosher salt

Combine the cream cheese, salmon, and butter in a food processor. Add the lemon juice, salt, and half the dill herb. Continue to blend until smooth. Spoon out portions of the mixture using a spoon so you have 6 evenly sized balls. Place on a tray and garnish with the leftover dill. Keep the tray in the fridge for 1 hour or until the mixture has become solidified.

Bacon and Egg Fat Bombs (10 servings total, 178 calories per serving, 19 grams fat, 1.0 grams carbs, 0 grams fiber, 1.0 grams net carbs)

a pinch of salt
a pinch of black pepper
2 hard-boiled eggs
.25 cup butter, grass-fed
4 medium slices of bacon
2.5 teaspoons mayonnaise

First, begin by setting your oven to 375 degrees F. On a parchment lined tray, lay out your bacon strips so you can bake for about 10 minutes in the oven until they are golden brown.

Remove from heat once crisp and brown in color. Crumble the pieces into smaller bite-size pieces once the bacon has cooled. Cut your hard-boiled eggs into small pieces. Dice your butter into smaller pieces and mix with the eggs in a large bowl. Add your salt and pepper seasoning and mayonnaise. Add any leftover bacon grease too! Be sure everything is well combined. Keep refrigerated for 15 minutes or until the mixture becomes colder. Remove from the fridge and use a cookie scoop to make about 10 balls. Roll each ball in the bacon pieces and place on a tray. Refrigerate the tray for 1 hour or until the mixture has solidified.

Parmesan Cheese Fat Bombs (10 servings total, 75 calories per serving, 7.1 grams fat, 3.0 grams carbs, 1.4 grams fiber, 1.6 grams net carbs)

5 ounces cream cheese, grass-fed
2 tablespoons parmesan cheese
a pinch of salt
6 olives, halved
1 teaspoon minced garlic

In a large bowl, mix the salt, garlic, olives, and cream cheese. Combine until well mixed. Use a cookie scoop to form 10 evenly sized balls and place on a lined baking sheet. Keep the tray refrigerated for 15 minutes or until the balls become more firm. Then roll each ball in the grated parmesan cheese until they are completely coated. Store the balls back in the fridge for 1 hour or until they have become solidified.

Meatball and Cheese Fat Bombs (8 servings total, 244 calories per serving, 26 grams protein, 28 grams fat, 4 grams carbs, 2 grams fiber, 2 grams net carbs)

.5 teaspoon kosher salt
.5 teaspoon paprika powder
1.5 teaspoon garlic powder
1 teaspoon butter or ghee for frying
2 cups ground beef, grass-fed
.75 cup mozzarella cheese
5 tablespoons parmesan cheese

Cut your mozzarella cheese into small cubes. They are going to be the cheesy center of your meatball! Combine the ground beef with the spices, parmesan cheese, and salt. Use a cookie scoop or tablespoon to make about 8 evenly sized balls. Take each ball of the beef mixture and flatten so you can place a few cubes of the mozzarella in the middle. Then form the meat back into a circle. In a skillet on medium heat, melt the butter or ghee for frying. Lightly pan fry the balls until they are golden brown.

Bacon Avocado Fat Bombs (6 servings total, 190 calories per serving, 18 grams fat, 2.9 grams carbs, 1.7 grams fiber, 1.2 grams net carbs)

4 tablespoons butter, grass-fed
.25 teaspoon red chili flakes
a pinch of salt
a pinch of black pepper
1 small ripe avocado, pitted and peeled
1 teaspoon minced garlic
5 medium pieces of bacon
1 teaspoon lemon or lime juice

First, preheat your oven to 350 degrees F. You can brown your bacon in the oven by spreading out the pieces on a lined baking sheet. Bake for 10-12 minutes until the pieces are golden brown. Remove from heat and crumble the pieces once they are cool. Keep the bacon grease! It will be added as an extra fat component to your fat bombs. In a medium size bowl, mash your avocado well to avoid any lumps. Mix with the softened butter and about half the bacon fat. Add your salt, pepper, garlic powder, lemon juice, and red chili flakes. Keep the bowl in the refrigerator for 15 minutes or until the mixture has become more firm. Remove from the fridge and use a cookie scoop to make 6 evenly sized balls. Dip each ball in the bacon pieces until they are well covered. Refrigerate again for 1 hour until the mixture has solidified.

Keto Pigs in a Blanket (4 servings total, 332 calories per serving, 7 grams carbs total, 27.9 grams fat, 1.9 grams fiber, 5.1 grams net carbs)

.75 cup almond flour
.25 teaspoon baking powder
.3 cup grated mozzarella cheese
.25 teaspoon salt
.5 teaspoon sesame seeds
1 large egg
.25 teaspoon garlic powder
4 medium hotdogs

Set your oven to 350 degrees F. Use the microwave to melt your mozzarella cheese on low until partly melted. Stir in the almond flour and egg until everything is well combined. Add baking powder, garlic powder, and salt and pepper to your mixture. Stir until the mixture forms a consistency like dough. Split into 12 pieces and spread each piece until it forms a flat oval. Place on a baking sheet. Cut each hotdog into 3 equal pieces. Place each piece in the piece of dough and wrap the dough around it. Sprinkle each piece with a few sesame seeds. Bake for 15-18 minutes or until the top of the dough turns golden brown.

Pizza Fat Bombs (8 servings total, 102 calories per serving, 9.6 grams fat, 4.0 grams carbs, 1.9 grams fiber, 2.1 grams net carbs)

8-10 black olives, pitted and sliced
.5 teaspoon salt
.5 teaspoon black pepper
3 teaspoons fresh basil or dried basil
15-20 slices pepperoni
1 cup cream cheese, grass-fed
3 tablespoons low-carb tomato pesto

First, cut your olives and pepperoni into small bite-size pieces. In a medium size bowl, mix together your tomato pesto, basil, and cream cheese. Add your salt and pepper seasoning, olives, and pepperoni. Use a cookie scoop or spoon to portion out 8 equal sized balls. You can garnish with any leftover basil or olives. Place the balls on a tray and refrigerate for 1 hour or until the mixture has solidified.

Sausage and Ricotta Cheese Fat Bombs (12 servings total, 60 calories per serving, 1 gram fat, 7 grams carbs, 0.6 grams fiber, 6.4 grams net carbs)

2/3 cup ricotta cheese
.5 teaspoon dried thyme
.25 teaspoon black pepper
.25 teaspoon dried oregano

.25 teaspoon paprika powder
.25 teaspoon dried parsley
.25 teaspoon kosher salt
1 pound pork sausage
.5 cup parmesan cheese
1 cup baby spinach
1 egg beaten
2 packages (~14 ounces) of low-carb pre-made pizza dough

First, set your oven to 400 degrees F. Prepare your pizza dough by dividing it into 12 evenly sized pieces of dough. In a skillet on low heat, cook your sausage with all the spice seasonings. Cook until golden brown for about 8-10 minutes and crumble the pieces. Add spinach, half the parmesan cheese, and ricotta cheese to the meat. Stir until the spinach is wilted and soft. Remove from heat and allow the mixture to cool.

Everything Bagel Fat Bombs (12 servings total, 40 calories per serving, 4 grams fat, 1.1 grams net carbs, 1 gram protein)

1 tablespoon butter, grass-fed, softened
.5 cup cream cheese, grass-fed, softened
.25 cup bagel seasoning

Make sure your butter and cream cheese are softened to room temperature. Mix them together until well combined using a hand mixer. Use a cookie scoop to make 12 evenly sized balls. Dip each ball into the bagel seasoning so it is fully coated. Place on a lined tray and keep the tray in the fridge for 1 hour or until the balls have solidified.

Sesame Seed Fat Bombs (6 servings total, 272 calories per serving, 29.4 grams fat, 1 gram carbs, 0 grams fiber, 1 gram net carbs)

.5 cup butter, grass-fed, softened
.5 teaspoon black pepper
.5 teaspoon salt
2 tablespoons sesame oil
2 teaspoons sesame seeds
.25 teaspoon red chili flakes

In a small saucepan on low heat, toast your sesame seeds until they turn light brown. This happens very quickly so be sure you're watching carefully so they don't burn! Remove from heat once golden brown. In a large bowl, mix your butter, sesame oil, salt and pepper seasonings, and red chili flakes until well combined. Refrigerate the mixture for 15 minutes or until the mixture becomes more firm. Then use a cookie scoop to form 6 evenly sized balls about 2 inches in size. Roll each ball in the toasted sesame seeds until it is well covered. Place on a tray and refrigerate the tray for 1 hour or until the mixture becomes solidified.

Jalapeno Popper Fat Bombs (10 servings total, 208 calories per serving, 4 grams protein, 20 grams fat, 2 grams carbs, 1 gram fiber, 1 gram net carbs)

.25 cup butter, grass-fed
2 medium-sized jalapeno peppers
.3 cup cheddar cheese, grated
4 ounces cream cheese, grass-fed, softened
5 medium slices of bacon

Set your oven to 325 degrees F. First, you want to ensure your peppers are de-seeded and chopped into fine pieces. Be sure to wash your hands after you are done! In a food processor, blend together the butter and cream cheese. You want to bake your bacon on a parchment paper lined baking sheet for 10-15 minutes depending on the thickness of the slices. Remove from heat once the pieces have turned crisp and golden brown. Crumble the bacon into pieces once it has cooled. In a medium size bowl, add the bacon grease, jalapeno peppers, and cheddar cheese and mix well. Then add the butter and cream cheese mixture and combine until everything is well incorporated. Place the bowl of mixture in the fridge for 15 minutes or until the mixture has become firm. Use a cookie scoop to make 10 equal sized balls. Dip each ball into the crumpled bacon pieces until well coated. Place the bacon-coated balls on a tray and keep refrigerated for 1 hour or until the mixture has solidified.

Butter Burger Fat Bombs (10 servings total, 125 calories per serving, 8 grams protein, 2.1 grams carbs, 1.1 grams fiber, 1 gram net carbs)

4 tablespoons butter, grass-fed, softened
.25 cup cheddar cheese, grated
a pinch of salt
a pinch of black pepper
.25 teaspoon garlic powder
1 pound ground beef, grass-fed

First, set your oven to 375 degrees F. In a large bowl, mix your ground beef with the salt and pepper seasoning and the garlic powder. Have a muffin tray lined with paper or silicone liners ready. Add 1 spoonful of the ground beef mixture into each liner and press well. You want to only use HALF the ground beef mixture! Then on top of the ground beef, you want to add a dollop of the softened butter. Go back and add a final spoonful of ground beef on top of the butter. Flatten with the spoon. Bake for 8-10 minutes or until the top layer of beef becomes golden brown.

Chapter 4:

The Keto Flu

What is the Keto Flu?

The keto diet has become so popular in recent years, but it can take some getting used to! Followers of the diet have coined the term "keto flu" to describe the initial symptoms a person might feel when they first begin a ketogenic diet. As your body adapts to a new diet with a drastic change in carbohydrates intake, the symptoms are very similar to the flu. It's almost like your body is going into withdrawal as it struggles to adjust to the change in the amount of carbohydrates you're taking in. Just like withdrawal is common when quitting addictive substances like tobacco or caffeine, it can also occur with carbs! As your body goes from burning sugar for energy to burning fat, it puts you through the wringer along the way.

The signs of the keto flu usually show up within the first few days a person has cut back on carbs on the keto diet. It generally kicks in between 24 and 48 hours as your body notices the cut in carbs. Symptoms can be mild or severe — it really depends from person to person. Some people might be able to transition to a keto diet without any symptoms. Other people may need a few weeks for their body to adjust. People who were used to eating more carbs and sugars in their diet could have a more difficult time adjusting and experience more symptoms compared to someone who already ate healthily and avoided carbs.

Think of this way — the average person's diet is composed of nearly 50-60% carbohydrates. They're cheap, easy, and quick to eat. When cutting that ratio all of a sudden to ~5%, the body is sure to have some trouble transitioning from that high-carb, low-fat diet to a low-carb, high-fat one. Factors like your physical health, water intake, genetics, and previous diet all can determine whether you will get the keto flu and how severe your symptoms might be.

Some of the symptoms include nausea, vomiting, constipation, diarrhea, weakness, muscle cramps, stomach pain, poor concentration or focus, difficulty sleeping, dizziness, and sugar cravings.

The good news is that these symptoms don't last very long! It'll only be until your body adjusts to the keto diet and is able to manage the change in macronutrients. It can be from a few days to a few weeks, maybe a month at maximum. If it lasts longer than that or symptoms don't seem to ease despite you eating the correct macro count, be sure to see a doctor for advice.

Still, the symptoms can be disheartening and overwhelming to newcomers on the diet and make you want to give up. But you want to keep in mind that it's only for a short period of time and that the benefits of a keto diet that you'll experience as you go with it will make up for a rough week or two at the beginning.

Why Do We Get the Keto Flu?

We've mentioned how the presence and the severity of the keto flu symptoms can depend on each individual person. Their previous carbs consumption, diet, and lifestyle all play a factor. If you ate a diet low in carbs and sugars, then you might only experience mild symptoms at having your carb intake cut further. If you had a diet high in carbs and sugars, then you can expect more severe symptoms of the keto flu, especially as your body experiences withdrawals from sugar.

What does the research say about why the keto flu occurs as you embark on the diet? Here are some of the top reasons why you experience these symptoms.

Water and sodium are flushed out of the body when you begin the diet. When you've cut the amount of carbs in your diet, there are fewer glycogen molecules being formed for the body to use those sugars as a fuel source. Insulin is normally used by the body to move sugars around the bloodstream, but with a reduced carb count, insulin levels in the body drop too. This signals your kidneys to release sodium from the body and that's how you end up losing water weight in the beginning stage of the keto diet. Studies have found some people can lose up to 10 pounds in water weight during the first 5 days alone!

Simply put, glycogen molecules that the body would have produced with carbohydrates are stored with about 3 grams of water each. On your first day of the keto diet, your main fuel source becomes the stored glycogen since you are no longer consuming carbs. This means almost a pound of water loss! With the body urinating more frequently and losing water and sodium, symptoms of nausea, cramping, dizziness, and headaches can occur. Research shows that just losing 2.8% of your body weight in water loss can impair your cognitive function. And a mere 2% loss in body weight can interfere with you physically. That's why signs of dehydration are so important to look out for. You can try and counteract the symptoms of dehydration by replenishing your fluid intake and adding a little extra salt in your meals.

Levels of the thyroid hormone T3 decrease. One study found that cutting carbohydrates completely from the test group's diet led to a 47% decrease in the T3 hormone. This is very important because T3 is the most important thyroid hormone that our body produces. Fewer amounts of it are produced than the T4 hormone, but it is more active in its role in the thyroid gland. It regulates the body's metabolism, basal temperature, and heart rate! Further studies found that the level of T3 hormone decreased if subjects consumed less than 120 grams of carbohydrates a day. It can vary from person to person but it's clear that this hormone is closely linked with the presence of carbohydrates in the body. Low amounts of T3 are linked with fatigue and difficulty concentrating or focusing.

The presence of the stress hormone cortisol in the body increases. With the cut in carbohydrates, your body feels it's under stress and starvation. It triggers a rush of hormones into the bloodstream including the stress hormone known as cortisol. This causes symptoms like irritability, mood swings, migraines, and difficulty sleeping. Research studies found that a lower carbohydrate intake diet also decreased levels of the hormone testosterone in men compared to a diet with high carbohydrates intake. Even though you have chosen to decrease carbohydrates, the body reacts to the change in diet as a stressor and produces cortisol. The good news is that your body will adjust to ketosis and your hormones will become stable again!

How to Fight the Keto Flu

The keto flu can be tough to fight when you're feeling so optimistic about starting the keto diet. But we have some tips to help you fight the flu and get through the symptoms to enjoy the benefits of a keto lifestyle!

Start slow: If you're having trouble adjusting to the drastic reduction of carbohydrates, you can always begin to eliminate them gradually over the period of a week or two. Slowly cutting back can help reduce your symptoms of the keto flu and helps you adjust to the keto lifestyle better. If you know that your diet was mostly composed of carbs, not to mention your high sugar intake, it might be better to start slowly and decrease your carb intake over a matter of days or weeks. This gives your body some time to adjust to lower cabs before you restrict it by going full keto.

Stay hydrated: Drinking enough water is necessary for any person no matter if they're dieting or not, but it can help you restore your water supply if you're on the keto diet. That's because the initial burst of weight loss on a keto diet is mostly water weight. The carbohydrates you would normally eat would create glycogen molecules for storage. But when you've reduced your carbs intake, glycogen levels plummet as water excretes from the body. That can put you at risk of dehydration if you aren't staying hydrated as you start the diet. You want to be sure you are drinking enough water to help with symptoms like fatigue and muscle cramps. Doctors highly suggest drinking at least 16-20 ounces of water per pound you are losing on the keto diet. Weigh yourself on the first day and track your weight loss to ensure you know how many pounds you're shedding.

Avoid strenuous exercise: We will have a whole chapter about exercising on a keto diet and how that helps you lose weight you want to get rid of. We'll give you ideas of exercises and how strength training is a great way to tone your body and develop muscle on a keto diet. But, it all happens in time! You do not want to dive right into stressful exercises when your body is adjusting to the keto diet. It's not recommended as you are fighting off symptoms of weakness, fatigue, or muscle cramps and can cause severe injury. Without enough carbohydrates, your performance will suffer and you need to give your body enough time to adjust to following the path of ketosis. Starting your rigorous workouts too early can make your symptoms worse. More leisure activities like yoga or walking can be done, but you want to put a pause on CrossFit, heavy weightlifting, or intense aerobic workouts until your body adapts to the keto diet.

Do yoga or light exercises: We've already said cut the high-intensity workouts until your keto flu passes but being physically active could help ease your symptoms. Even just taking a walk around the neighborhood will increase your fat burning and push your body towards ketosis. It will help clear the brain fog and give you more mental acuity. If you feel worse, be sure you stop and check that you aren't dehydrated and that you've eaten enough fat. Yoga or breathing exercises are a great way to regulate your thoughts and relieve stress as well. Your cortisol levels will already be high during this keto flu period as your body adjusts to the cut in carbs. Taking some time for a light physical activity like walking, yoga, or stretching will be nice to shift your focus.

Make sure you're eating enough fat (and carbs): When starting the keto diet, the cut in carbs can make you feel restricted and leave you craving the forbidden items (cookies, pasta, bread, bagels, sugar... and more!). To cure those hunger pains and leave you feeling fuller, you need to be sure you're eating enough fat which makes up the majority of your macronutrients. You're not supposed to go low carb *AND* low fat like some diets — its low carb and HIGH fats! High-quality fats will now be your major fuel source to help your body produce ketones for energy. Be sure you're tracking your macros and calorie intakes when you first start the keto diet to ensure you're eating enough and eating the right things. A quick way to consume some high-quality fats is by making fat bombs, the popular term coined for keto-friendly snacks that can be sweet or savory and quickly increase your macro count for the day. If you're not eating fats then you run the risk of stalling your weight loss and feeling tired or hungry.

Electrolytes: Replacing the body's electrolyte losses is another way to fight symptoms of the keto flu. When following a keto diet, the levels of insulin in the body decrease. When that happens, the kidneys release excess sodium. To ensure your body is getting enough salt and electrolytes, use regular iodized table salt in your meals and in water. Himalayan pink salt is a great addition to your diet and has more than 80 minerals! Increasing your salt intake will counteract the water loss. Some ketogenic researchers state that you should include an extra 5 to 8 grams of salt (1-1.5 teaspoon) in your diet the first week you start the diet because of the loss in water weight that's to come. Sodium, iodine, and potassium are very important for your body so you want to be sure you are replenishing your body with the nutrients it needs. Bone broth is a great dish to get electrolytes like potassium and sodium while being hydrating at the same time. Foods high in potassium like salmon, nuts, avocados, and leafy green vegetables should be eaten a lot too. Magnesium is also a very important mineral that improves your quality of sleep and treats muscle cramps. Some people recommend taking a magnesium supplement if you are having muscle aches or pains when starting keto.

Recommended Doses:		
Sodium	5 to 7 grams iodized salt per day	Table salt, Himalayan pink salt
Magnesium	400 grams per day (men) 310 grams per day (women)	Chicken, beef, fish, spinach, or a magnesium supplement
Potassium	3,500 milligrams per day	Fish, meat, squash, pumpkins, leafy greens

Get enough sleep: If you're struggling with the keto diet, you want to be sure you're getting rest to allow your body a smoother transition. Getting at least 7-9 hours of sleep a night is important. As your body is experiencing changes in its diet and switching fuel sources, sleep can help reduce your fatigue and stress. The body increases the amount of stress hormones in the bloodstream as it adjusts to the keto diet and you want to counteract that by remaining stress-free and having enough rest at night. When you have issues on getting adequate sleep, try a magnesium supplement which is a necessary nutrient for the body anyway. Try a power nap throughout the day if you can't manage a full 7 hours of sleep a night. Have a routine at the end of the day to go from work mode to sleep mode. Try to avoid screens, make sure your bedroom is dark and quiet, and have a cup of tea... whatever you need to do to sleep well!

Take some ketone supplements: These are additional ketone salts you can add to your diet to urge your body towards ketosis. They provide your body with extra ketones so it becomes more adapted to burning fat instead of sugar. This can be helpful for people who are struggling with the diet and can even eliminate symptoms of the keto flu. Supplementing your diet with MCT oil can also help. This oil is made of high-quality fat triglycerides which is what the body is going to be burning as an energy source instead of carbs. If you take some MCT oil, it will go directly to your liver and be converted into ketones to push your body towards ketosis. It can help some people fight against symptoms of keto flu to feel more energetic quicker.

Be patient: If you've committed to the keto diet then you're probably eager to see the results of weight loss and overall improved health. Suffering through the keto flu can feel disappointing as you're stuck feeling lethargic and too weak to exercise like you'd wanted to. The important thing is to follow the tips mentioned above and be patient with yourself. As we've described at the beginning of the book, your body is following a different pathway to produce the energy you need. The cut in carbs reduces the amount of glycogen sugar molecules produced and your body will instead enter ketosis to burn fat molecules for fuel. The keto flu is just a beginning hurdle to get through! Symptoms will subside as your body becomes adjusted to ketosis and a new fuel source. Take time to rest, don't stress over things you can't control, hydrate, and double check that you're eating enough fats and following the keto macro guidelines. Once this hump is over, you'll be achieving your healthy eating goals on a keto diet!

Up your carb intake if necessary: If you're still struggling, you may need to up your carbohydrates intake in order to ease your symptoms of the keto flu. This will help you feel better and give your body a chance to adjust to burning fat. It will help you feel more energized physically and help you focus mentally. Your goal should still be to minimize your carbs and follow the standard keto diet though. You can slowly adjust your diet and cut out those carbs as you plan your meals and find substitutes to the foods you enjoy. Working towards the 5% macronutrient carb count should still be your goal to produce definitive weight loss results and improve your health overall.

Chapter 5:

Exercising on a Keto Diet

Exercising on Keto

Exercising and working out on a keto diet is absolutely possible and encouraged to help you accelerate your weight loss. The keto diet itself is designed to help you lose the stubborn fat you haven't been able to get rid of. Following a keto diet coupled with exercise will help you lose more significant weight and lose that weight faster. It's not necessary and you will still lose weight and gain the health benefits with just following the diet, but following an exercise routine will speed up your weight loss if you have a weight goal in mind.

Before starting your exercise routine, it is important to first understand how your body processes the energy you need and what limitations in exercises that could mean. When first adjusting to the keto diet, the lack of carbs can make you seem groggy or tired. You're going through the "keto flu" as we described in Chapter 4. You can feel weak or lethargic and wonder how you'll ever find the energy to exercise. The good news is that these symptoms only last a few weeks until your body adjusts to the natural process of using ketones for energy instead of carbohydrates like it has been used to. It will begin to harness energy through the high-quality fats you're eating instead of the low-quality carbs of before. As your body begins to adjust to ketosis, you'll find that your energy levels will return to normal and you are able to focus on exercising.

First, it's important to realize which exercises would be impacted by your keto diet. If you have an exercise that requires maximum effort from your muscles for more than 10 seconds, the muscles begin to rely on glucose sugar molecules for energy. When you restrict carbs, your muscle cells will crave sugar for energy for those high-intensity activities. Activities that require that effort for more than 10 seconds to 2 minutes will be impacted. That includes things like:

- lifting heavy weights for more than a few reps
- playing sports that have minimal break times like soccer or rugby
- high-intensity interval training like CrossFit
- sprinting or swimming for longer than 10 seconds like the 50- or 100-meter swim.

That's not a complete list but it gives you an idea of what type of activities and workouts could be affected. It depends on the person — some people might be able to last 30 seconds while others burn out and feel fatigue in 10 or 15 seconds. It's important that you know your limit and be careful as not to jeopardize your health.

Now, in order to exercise regularly while being on this diet, it is extremely necessary for you to have the right amount of macronutrients on your keto diet. Eating the right amounts of fat and protein becomes even more important because that's what will help you gain muscle mass and keep your energy levels up when exercising.

- **Protein**: Protein is key for many bodily functions that carbs and fats cannot do. It's very important for muscle building and burning calories. When you are not consuming an adequate amount of protein, then you will lose muscle mass which can increase your body fat percentage. While following keto, it's important that you have multiple sources of protein intake and divide them throughout the day after your workouts to boost your energy after exercising. Fish, meat, eggs, high-quality dairy products are great sources of protein and you can even get low-carb protein powders. Researchers at the Society of Sports Nutrition state that a protein intake of 1 gram per pound of body mass (1.4-2 grams per kilogram) is the ideal amount for athletes who exercise regularly.

- **Carbs**: Generally, a keto diet will want you to limit your carbs intake to 35 grams or less a day. But if you are a more active person or an athlete that plays high-intensity sports, you might have to increase the amount of carbs to improve your performance. To do this, you can either increase your carb intake by following the advice of keto researchers. Follow a more targeted keto diet where you consume an amount of carbs prior to exercise or include 1-2 "re-feeding" days in your week where carbs are allowed to help you store up your energy. That's an extreme option because it will make it more difficult for you to achieve ketosis, but it might be the option for professional athletes or those who are training for an event.

- **Fat**: The right amount of fat is very important when following a keto diet. If you eat too much, your body will not make enough energy and you'll lose weight because you're starving yourself. If you eat too much, you'll gain weight. It's very important that you monitor your daily fat intake to ensure 70-75% of your daily calories are coming from high-quality fats. You can tweak this number a little depending on your weight goals. Do you want to gain weight? Then you should slightly increase your fat intake by 250-500 calories. Do you want to lose weight? Then you want to decrease your fat calories until you are 250-500 calories at a deficit. The number of calories you go down by should be even higher if you are obese or overweight and want to see serious progress in your weight loss.

It's very important to realize that high-intensity workouts that push the body will need to utilize burning sugar at some point in the workout. The more you push your body and want to have a "harder" workout, the more your body will want to fall back on using sugar molecules for quick fuel. One study found that in an exercise conducted on race walking, participants on a low carb diet took an average of 24 seconds longer to complete the race. Participants on a high carb diet or more of a cyclical keto diet that includes feeding days performed better at the race. Well, you might wonder why that is the case with simply walking? But keep in mind race walking is different than simply taking a nice walk around the block after dinner. It requires athletes to push their bodies to have the best performance and time for conquering the race distance. If they don't have enough sugars available, then their performance will decrease.

It is important to note that other scientific studies show that keto-adapted athletes may not experience a decrease in their performance. Once athletes become adapted to their keto diet and are consistently burning more fat than carbs for energy, their body lets them use more glycogen when they need to increase their intensity in a workout. So, it is possible for athletes to adapt to a keto lifestyle. But with high-intensity sports with few timeouts like tennis, rugby, soccer, and lacrosse, it's more likely performance will be impacted negatively. These sports place a higher energy demand on the body which means the body will require more glycogen than it has by following a keto diet. These athletes should consult a diet coach to see how they can tweak their keto diet by including some carb feeding days throughout the week or increasing their daily carb limit. When it comes to athletes of other sports like football, golf, boxing or wrestling, they can follow the ketogenic diet without experiencing deficiencies in performance. Because the high-intensity workout time for these sports is usually around or less than 10 seconds, their bodies rely on the ATP phosphate pathway to create energy for use. Weightlifters, wrestlers, and boxers can especially utilize the keto diet to shed water weight so they can tone their muscle mass. A lot of athletes will utilize the keto weight during the offseason of their sports. Let's be honest, without regular workouts or games and enjoying an unhealthy diet, athletes will need some help trimming that excess weight before training begins! The keto diet is a great way for them to do that because it helps them lose weight without losing any muscle mass.

CARDIO: When it comes to low to moderate intensity cardio workouts, you will find the keto diet does not impair your performance. You might even be able to work out for longer while you are in ketosis! For moderate physical activity, a person's heart rate is about 50 to 70% of their maximum heart rate. To find your maximum heart rate, you subtract your age from 220. For example, if someone is 40 years old, their estimated maximum heart rate would be 220 - 40 = 180 beats per minute. To find the 50% and 70% levels of that, you would do the math to find: 50% level: 180 x .50 = 90 beats per minute, 70% level = 180 x .70 = 126 beats per minute. This gives athletes on a keto diet an idea of where their heart rate should fall when performing cardio workouts. As you are adjusting to the keto diet and beginning your workouts, aim for the 50% level. Once you adjust and feel your energy level has stabilized, you can maintain a higher heart rate without needing to feed on too many carbs.

Here are some examples of low to moderate intensity cardio workouts you can perform after you've gotten over the keto flu and your energy levels have adjusted to the keto diet.

- aerobic training classes
- swimming
- cycling
- running
- walking
- interval training classes
- yoga
- Pilates
- recreational sports that have breaks in between

It's important to note that even a low to moderate intensity aerobic cardio workout will exercise your muscles and help you on your way to losing weight. You should not put yourself at risk by attempting high-intensity workouts or sports like lacrosse, soccer, or tennis that do not have enough breaks.

Simply taking a short walk around the neighborhood can be a great way to exercise without taxing your body as you get adjusted to the keto diet. As your body adjusts to ketosis and you feel your energy level has returned to normal, you can perform some of the other aerobic workouts mentioned above. Those workouts use up more of your energy. Be patient with yourself because your body is adjusting to extracting energy from a new pathway and using fat for its fuel source. High-intensity workouts should be scaled back until you feel your energy level can meet up with the demands of your exercise.

Low to moderate intensity cardio workouts are great and encouraged to help you lose weight!

WEIGHTLIFTING: Are you looking to become stronger and increase your muscle mass? Does your workout routine contain a strength training routine? Then the keto diet works perfectly for you! Weightlifting is one of those exercises where your body doesn't require glucose for energy because the quick muscular actions usually don't last more than 10 seconds. That means the body can rely on stored ATP molecules instead of needing an intake of carbs. What does this mean? It means your light to moderate weightlifting routine will not be negatively impacted! Research shows that as long as you are using the appropriate amount of weight and increasing that volume slightly every week, you can still have muscle growth. It's all about following a muscle building program as a guide while you follow your keto routine. A study found that in a group of men who followed a weight lifting program, the ones on a keto diet showed more of a muscle mass increase after the final week of the testing period. Now, if you want to follow it with higher reps and lighter weights, then you might have to supplement your diet with extra carbs as we mentioned above.

Pre and Post Workout

Pre Workout: Workout smoothies to take before exercising are very popular but it can be difficult to find ones that have the effective dosage of supplements for you. Though these smoothies even the keto-friendly ones will contain performance boosting supplements, they are not going to be tailor-made for your needs or contain enough of a dose that you see improvements. In order to make a smoothie perfect for your needs, we urge you to make them yourself and invest in the supplements that work for you. Protein powder, taurine, exogenous ketones, and MCTs can all be added to a keto-friendly smoothie to give you a boost of energy.

If you need some help to boost your exercise performance, there are some low carb or no carb keto-friendly supplements that you can take.

- **Protein Powder**: You should try to get most of your protein from food sources but using protein powder is a great way to meet your protein demands. Adding some of this powder to your smoothies is a great way to boost your energy before a workout. Stick with complete protein powders like whey, collagen, or casein.

    Suggestion: Add about 20-40 grams of the powder to your smoothies before or after a workout to stimulate muscle cell reactions.

- **Creatine**: This is the most researched supplement that works to more effectively increase the output of your body's phosphate system. This supplement is great for weightlifters.

Suggestion: Taking 5 grams per day is a great way to increase your body's muscle mass.

- **Medium Chain Triglycerides (MCTs):** This is a type of saturated fat that goes straight to your liver to be converted into ketones. MCTs are a great way to push your body into ketosis right when you need it before a round of cardio or endurance exercises.

    Suggestion: Take about 1-2 tablespoons of MCT powder or oil before your workouts for a jolt of energy.

- **Exogenous Ketones:** This ketone powder is composed of chemical salts and esters and provides the body with instant energy. However, this powder can be dangerous and conflict with the liver's natural ketone production so it should be taken with MCTs.

    Suggestion: Try using an exogenous ketone salt to boost your energy before working out. Take with MCTs for better ketone production.

- **Taurine**: This is a type of organic acid that has been found to improve exercise performance in athletes even more than caffeine which the body can become adapted to. Research shows participants in a cycling experiment who consumed taurine were better able to fight their fatigue and had increased power during their cycling sprint.

    Suggestion: Start with 50 milligrams of taurine per kilogram of your body mass but work to decrease that number until you find an amount where you can get the same effects.

- **Beta-alanine**: This is a substance found very commonly in pre-packaged pre-workout smoothies. It tends to give you a tingling sensation in your body but athletes say they can do two to three more reps in the gym when weightlifting after taking beta-alanine.

    Suggestion: Take 2-5 grams of beta-alanine every day. Pair it with 5 grams of creatine every day to get better results in the gym. If you're uncomfortable with the tingling sensation, decrease it to 1 gram taken 2-4 times a day.

- **L-Citrulline**: This is a substance well known to athletes who use it to increase their aerobic and anaerobic sports performance. It's been shown to improve endurance if taken before a workout.

    Suggestion: Take 6,000-8,000 milligrams about an hour before an intense workout training.

- **Fish Oil**: Fish oil supplements have become popular because of the special omega 3 fatty acids that help muscle synthesis and increase brain activity. The American Heart Association recommends at least 1 gram of DHA and EPA fatty acids daily. That's about a 3 ounce serving of fish or sardines a day or you can take an over the counter fish oil supplement.

    Suggestion: Take at least 1 gram a day.

Post Workout: Previous research used to urge athletes to slam their system with protein shakes right after a workout to encourage muscle growth. Instead, new research shows that muscle growth happens about 4-6 hours after eating protein.

For example, if you had 30 grams of protein powder before a workout, your body works to create new muscle growth for about 4-6 hours as it synthesizes the powder. That's why it's important to maintain your protein count on a keto diet and have protein every 4-6 hours. Have your biggest protein meal after working out to boost muscle growth and recovery. Fish would be the perfect meal to have because it's a source of protein and rich in omega 3 fatty acids.

Smoothie Recipes

Here we have some pre-workout smoothie recipes for you to enjoy before hitting the gym! Just add your ingredients to your blender and mix until smooth! You'll feel a boost in your endurance and energy levels and notice better performance during your workouts.

Keto-friendly Citrus Green Smoothie (1 serving total, 207 calories, 20 grams fat, 2 grams fiber, 5 grams carbs, 3 grams protein, 3 grams net carbs)

.5-1 tablespoon lemon zest
.5-1 tablespoon orange zest
.5-1 tablespoon lime zest
8 ounces almond milk
a handful of ice
5-8 drops Stevia liquid sweetener
1 tablespoon keto-friendly MCT oil

Keto Strawberry Milkshake (1 serving total, 368 calories, 39 grams fat, 2 grams fiber, 4 grams carbs, 2 grams net carbs, 1.7 grams protein)

.75 cup full-fat coconut milk
a handful of ice
.25 cup heavy whipping cream
2 tablespoons Stevia liquid sweetener
.5 cup strawberries, fresh or frozen
1-2 tablespoons MCT oil

Blackberry Chocolate Shake (1 serving total, 346 calories, 35 grams fat, 12 grams carbs, 7 grams fiber, 2.7 grams protein, 5 grams net carbs)

.25 cup blackberries, fresh or frozen
1 cup unsweetened full-fat coconut milk
a handful of ice
2 tablespoons unsweetened cocoa powder
10-12 drops Stevia liquid sweetener
1-2 tablespoons MCT oil

Cucumber Spinach Smoothie (1 serving total, 330 calories, 32 grams fat, 6 grams carbs, 2 grams fiber, 3 grams net carbs, 10 grams protein)

2 handfuls of spinach
2.5 ounces cucumber, peeled and diced
a handful of ice
1 cup full-fat coconut milk
10-12 drops Stevia liquid sweetener
1-2 tablespoons MCT oil

Keto Tropical Smoothie (1 serving total, 355 calories, 32 grams fat, 7 grams carbs, 3 grams fiber, 4 grams net carbs, 4 grams protein)

a handful of ice
.25 cup sour cream
.75 cup unsweetened full-fat coconut milk
1 tablespoon MCT oil
2 tablespoons flaxseed
.25 teaspoon mango extract
.25 teaspoon banana extract

Chapter 6:

Tips to Get You Started & Mistakes to Avoid!

Tips to Embrace a Keto Lifestyle

If you are deciding to take some steps, there are some steps you should take to help yourself along the way. These tips can help you start your diet on the right note to ensure your success — whether that's in losing weight or becoming healthier overall.

Get rid of the temptations! Goodbye carbs, soda, and sugar! Let's be honest — carbs are tempting! If you have them around, you might be tempted to have some. If you keep your usual carbohydrates in stock, you might be tempted to keep eating them. To begin your keto diet, first, you should clear out all of the carbohydrates you can from your kitchen. Pasta, cereal, snacks, processed foods... it might sound extreme but those are the rules! It's also important that you're aware of your daily sugar intake. It might just be a spoon of sugar in your morning coffee, dessert at lunch, maybe a handful of cookies as a snack in the evening... it all adds up! And all of those will need to be cut from your diet when going keto. If you're serious about keto, start cutting back on your sugar intake now. Diet soda is also detrimental to the keto diet because it uses sugar substitutes that fool your brain into increasing your blood sugar. When you get rid of all the temptations, you'll be astonished at how much room there is in your pantry! But that is the space that you can fill up now with healthy ingredients to help you go far on a keto lifestyle!

Incorporate healthy vegetables and protein into your diet. As you're studying about the keto diet, you're becoming familiar with the list of "allowed" items. You should become familiar with the list of what vegetables to eat. Mostly it's the above ground, non-starchy, leafy green vegetables that are keto approved. If you're not already a veggie lover, then try some new ones! Spinach, kale, broccoli, cabbage... whether it's lightly sautéed or grilled or in a smoothie form, try these new foods to get an idea of what you will be eating on a keto diet. Try different recipes to see what type of cooking appeals to you and fits with your busy schedule. The same goes for protein sources. If you have mostly been a meat lover, try fish and poultry. Fish are known to be rich in omega 3 fatty acids and can be the perfect keto-friendly dinner option.

Invest in a food scale or measuring tools. As a keto beginner, weighing the food you eat and being aware of portion sizes is going to be key. Invest in a food scale so you feel confident when weighing your food for new recipes. This will help you avoid overeating. Also, be sure you have proper measuring spoons and cups to help you with trying all your new keto-friendly recipes. A difference between one teaspoon and tablespoon when measuring can mean hundreds of extra calories!

Keep keto friendly snacks on hand. This tends to be a common pitfall for busy people on a keto diet. They might not prep or plan ahead of time and at the end of a busy day, they're tempted to break their diet. No matter how good your intentions to follow your diet, if you follow through on an unhealthy carb-loaded dinner at the end of a long day, you've ruined your macro count for the day! Be sure you've stocked your pantry with filling snacks like deli meats, beef jerky, eggs, and keto-friendly fruits and veggies. Have more protein like bacon slices, beef jerky, and eggs. We've also included recipes for fat bombs that make a quick and filling snack!

Count your calories. When you first begin your keto diet, it's important you count your macros and your carbohydrates to ensure you're following the recommended guidelines. To begin, start counting your carbs throughout the day so you have an idea of how much you need to cut out. Don't forget hidden carbs! Look at the nutrition facts and be consciously aware of what you're eating. Calculate net carbs: Total carbs - Fiber = Net Carbs. There are many apps you can download to help you! You want to stay calorie deficit. Try and spread out your meals throughout the day so you are not overeating in a short time span.

Decrease the stress factors in your life. High levels of the stress hormone elevate your blood sugar and stop your body from effectively burning fat. A stressful lifestyle will actually send false hunger signals to your body and make you gain weight if you tend to overeat. When starting a keto lifestyle, it's important you're in the right period of your life to make the changes with enthusiasm. If you're going through a stressful time, then it might not be the right time to embark on a keto lifestyle that has such dramatic changes to your diet. Be sure that you're taking the time every day to decompress and let go of the stressors of the day. Whether that's exercising, yoga, meditation, or making sure you have a good night sleep, you want to take some time to relax.

Stay hydrated. Drinking enough water is an important part of staying healthy no matter what diet you're on. It's even more important with a keto lifestyle because having such a small amount of carbs will trigger you losing a lot of water weight. Generally, the rule is that you should drink half of your weight in ounces of water. So if you weigh 140 pounds, 140/2 = 70 ounces or about 8.75 glasses of an 8-ounce glass of water. If you're an athlete, you need to increase that number. Keep a bottle with you at all times so you can be drinking throughout the day.

Notice how your body reacts to dairy products. With the keto diet, there's sometimes whose bodies don't tolerate dairy well. That can cause health problems and impede your weight loss. Those people would need to adjust their diet as to substitute for dairy products. Be sure to notice how your body is reacting and if you're experiencing any lactose intolerant symptoms.

Be prepared for when you're eating out or at a friend's house. It can seem overwhelming if you're out at dinner and scrambling to find a keto-friendly option on the menu. But you can feel more confident if you know what to ask for. But it gets easier if you know exactly what to ask for. Get familiar with the list of approved keto items and feel free to ask for substitutes of more keto-friendly vegetables.

Educate yourself on a keto diet! Last but not least, it's important you know exactly what you're getting into. Like this book has aimed to educate you on so much related to the keto diet, it's important you are aware of what you can eat, what you can't, what types of exercise to perform, how to create keto-friendly recipes, and more! The more educated you are about the aspects of a keto lifestyle, the more confident you'll feel following one!

Common Mistakes on a Keto Diet

When talking about the keto diet, it's only natural we hit upon what are some common mistakes. These may seem like little mistakes, but they can greatly impact your calorie intake and maybe cause you to over or under eat. This can jeopardize your health so it's important you're aware of any possible mistakes to avoid them.

Being afraid of eating high-fat content. It can be hard for people who have tried other diets to get used to the idea of eating so much fat! That's what you're supposed to stay away from if you want to lose weight. But with keto, it's the other way around. If you're a beginner, you want to be sure you're counting your macros so you are indeed having 70-75% of your calories coming from high-quality fats. This is what will keep you full and give you the energy to get through the day. Try to buy healthy, organic fats and grass-fed items so you are consuming the best quality.

Not drinking enough water. As we mentioned above, when you first begin shedding pounds on the keto diet, it'll be mostly water weight. That means you need to stay hydrated with plenty of fluids and electrolytes. If you live in a warmer climate or are an athlete, then it's important you drink even more water.

Living a sedentary lifestyle. As detailed in Chapter 5, an active lifestyle coupled with the keto diet is the perfect formula to help you lose weight. If you're not incorporating some light physical activity to your routine, then you won't properly gain the benefits of keto. You don't have to be hitting the gym a few times a week — even light aerobic activity like walking for 15-20 minutes is great!

You're eating too much protein. Since you've cut back on carbs, it can be tempting to want to fill up your hunger with protein. But the truth is, eating much protein will have a negative effect on your keto lifestyle. You want to stick to the macro counts: 75% fat, 20% protein, ~5% carbs. Think of it this way — your body has a protein limit for each day. When you hit that limit, it stores the excess protein as fat! Count your calories or use an app to help you keep track of how much you're eating throughout the day. This keeps you aware of what type of foods you're consuming and ensuring you aren't hitting your protein limit.

You're not looking for hidden carbs. Even if you've been following a keto lifestyle for a few months, you might have relaxed about it and are missing some "hidden" carbs that are putting you over your daily carb limit. Things like condiments on meals or hidden sugars in snacks can halt your weight loss. It's important you double check the labels to ensure you're not missing the carbs count. Instead, use extra virgin olive oil as a salad dressing or butter that counts as a fat on your meats.

You're not eating a variety of foods to your diet. There are clear restrictions on the keto diet, but there are also so many foods you CAN eat! If you're eating the same bland foods for your meals, then chances are you'll become frustrated with the diet and be tempted by other foods not allowed. Try and experiment with new foods so that you find a new favorite! Every food has its nutrients of unique vitamins and minerals for you to gain through consumption. So, try new protein sources, veggies, and fat bombs as snacks. There are so many choices — sweet, chocolaty, savory, or ones packed with meat!

Obsessing over your weight. We know — that's easier said than done! Especially when you're anxious to see those pounds drop! But checking your weight over and over or agonizing why the diet isn't working yet will not motivate you and is not productive. Instead, focus on what you are eating and planning delicious keto-friendly meals that are within your macro count. Keep track of your calories and incorporate some physical activity into your day. Be patient as you wait for results and remember the overall health benefits you'll be gaining.

Motivational Work Out Tips!

If you're anxious about working out on a keto diet, here are some tips to get you started!

Don't start any new workouts when beginning a keto diet. This is not the time to suddenly increase your weights or add an extra mile to your run! The initial period of "keto flu" can make you feel sluggish or weak. The symptoms will pass as your body gets used to burning ketones instead of carbs, but you don't want to jeopardize your health or risk an accident by starting a new workout. Stick to what you're used to until you fall back to your normal energy level.

Give your body time to adjust. As we've illustrated in the book and dived into about the effect of keto flu, it's important that you give your body time to adjust to the keto lifestyle. Some people might be cutting more than half of their daily carbohydrate intake! It's okay to admit if you feel slow or weak for a few days. Skip a few workouts so you don't risk a chance of injury. Be patient with your body and know that it'll take anywhere from 2-10 days for ketosis to occur. That feeling will pass and you'll feel more energized to resume physical activity.

Skip high-intensity workouts until you are fully adjusted to keto. We detailed in Chapter 5 about how your high-intensity workout performances could be impaired on the keto diet. Glycogen is low and some workouts require sugar for energy instead of ketones. This depends from person to person, but you want to be sure of how you feel before starting any intense workouts. You want to wait until your energy level has fully returned to normal. If you need an extra burst of energy to get through your workouts, you can include a protein powder supplement to your pre-workout smoothies.

Make sure you're eating enough fat. It can be tough to get into the habit of eating a lot of fat content on a keto diet, but if you're not eating enough, you can actually lose muscle mass. Not to mention, you'll feel hungrier! You want to counterbalance the low carb count with a high intake of fat so you can push your body towards ketosis. Focus on eating quality fats like grass-fed cheeses, avocado, or extra virgin olive oil, and full-fat yogurt.

Don't under eat! If you aren't following keto correctly, then you could be damaging your body and potentially losing muscle mass. Especially if you are exercising, you want to be sure you are meeting your caloric limit. The keto diet requires you to eat healthy fats to quench your appetite. That's why counting your calories is so important! If you're counting calories, you could be under eating which will leave you deprived of energy and feeling constantly hungry.

Spread out your workouts. Don't attempt to do too much in one day! That's a taxing workout for anybody but especially if you're on the keto diet and need some time to replenish your calories. Spread out your workouts in the week so you don't feel fatigued or risk injury to yourself. Do light weightlifting 2-3 times a week and light cardio 2-3 times a week, but preferably not on the same days! You don't want to cause muscle damage or overexert yourself. Don't be ashamed to take a rest day! Your body needs rest to relax in order to burn weight and increase muscle growth.

Don't fill your diet with unnecessary calories. Some people believe that you need to have a protein shake before and after every workout. But new research shows that muscle growth actually occurs 4-8 hours after you've worked out and synthesized some form of protein. It's all about eating well throughout the day, not just focusing on your pre and post-workout routine!

Motivate yourself by remembering all the other aspects of working out. It can be frustrating sometimes if you're not losing weight fast enough, especially when you're working out and sacrificing such delicious things like carbs and sugar. On a keto diet, after you lose that first round of initial water weight, your weight loss might plateau as you near your goal weight. Remind yourself of all the health benefits involved with keto and exercising such as reducing your body's resistance to insulin, reducing stress, getting a good night's sleep, and lowering your risk of heart disease. Those are lasting benefits that will improve your overall quality of life!

Listen to your body and your doctor. The first weeks on a keto diet can be an adjustment as you're cutting your carbs count drastically. If you're feeling dizzy or tired even after a few weeks on the diet, it's important you keep track of your calories and avoid any strenuous physical activity. Talk to your doctor about how you're feeling and what you could be doing wrong. Your health is a priority!

Chapter 7:

Intermittent Fasting

What is Intermittent Fasting?

Fasting is a common term associated with religions, but it's not thought of as something to be implemented into your daily routine. But the truth is, fasting is an ancient tradition that is successful at helping you shed unwanted pounds and gain many benefits on a person's health. In fact, fasting intermittently is a way to prevent insulin resistance, lose weight, lower your blood pressure, and improve your overall concentration and mental alertness. Most of the research is focused on intermittent fasting or fasting on and off because that form has been shown to be much more successful in losing weight than other fad diets.

Some people will try to equate fasting with starvation. They will say that giving up food is extreme, that you're starving your body simply to lose weight. But that's not true at all! Starving yourself means you have involuntarily given up food and that you don't know where your next meal is coming from. Fasting is something you are doing voluntarily, knowing that you are healthy and able to complete the fast. It's something you're doing to lose weight or to gain other health benefits. Just like with the keto diet, how you guide your body to a cycle of burning fats and ketones instead of carbs — your body also begins to adjust while you are fasting to burn the energy you already have stored.

Intermittent fasting involves cycles of fasting, then eating, fasting, then eating again. How long does the fast last? That's completely up to you! The rules of intermittent fasting do not declare certain days or foods off limits. In fact, it encourages you to eat healthily and load your body with calories from carbohydrates, proteins, and fats to power through the fasting phase. You should not eat anything but you are allowed to have beverages like coffee, water, tea, and other non-caloric beverages. In fact, you're encouraged to have caffeine during your fast! Caffeine actually dulls the body's hunger pangs and makes you feel fuller. It's like how if you drink a few cups of coffee first thing in the morning, you're not hungry much later. It's a way to contain your growling stomach and make yourself feel full even if you're not gaining calories.

The goal in fasting is to allow the body to adapt without food for a set period of time so the body can utilize burning excess fat it has stored away. Fat is already food energy the body can use, but as you're continuing to feed yourself during the day, it uses the new fuel for energy instead of using the backup supply! Just like with the keto diet how the body is urged to use ketones for fuel instead of carbs, fasting for a short period of time guides the body to use the fat reserves it has stored away. The body will need fuel and with you abstaining from food, it will "turn on itself" and use what it already has!

The Health Benefits of Fasting

It sounds tough to be giving up food during the day. It's different than dieting because you're actually quitting cold turkey. But it's only for a set period of time and the benefits will surprise you. Scientific research proves that intermittent fasting has lots of health benefits that should be considered, especially for people who may be at risk for certain health conditions. Fasting regularly could help them. But even if you're not battling your health, it's a great way to lose weight and gain many benefits and become overall more alert and healthy.

You will lose weight! Sounds obvious — but this is the biggest attraction to people who are just not able to lose the pounds. Logically, if you're limiting the hours you are eating in the day, you will be eating less. This cuts down on the number of fattening snacks and high fructose syrup that you might be eating. By abstaining from all food, you're cutting down on the calories you're eating. And how does weight loss? Only if you're calorie deficit! A study showed that with test subjects of people on an intermittent fasting diet and one group on a traditional diet plan, the intermittent fasting group lost more weight after a year and regained less weight too. That's very important because you want to be able to keep the weight off!

It can lower your cholesterol. Cholesterol is divided into two parts — LDL (Low-Density Lipoprotein) or "bad cholesterol" and HDL (High-Density Lipoprotein) or "good cholesterol". Having high cholesterol increases a person's risk of heart disease and having a stroke or heart attack. Fasting is proven to decrease LDL or bad cholesterol. A study found that when participants fasted, their LDL levels decreased by almost 25%! Some participants were even able to decrease the dosage of their cholesterol medicine. The goal of fasting is to burn stored fat so the liver decreases the amount of cholesterol it produces which means your "bad cholesterol" levels decrease significantly.

It reduces your risk of diabetes. Diabetes is a disease that is due to the body's miscommunication with the insulin it creates to process your body's glucose molecules. Fasting does not alter the concentration of glucose molecules, but it improves your body's sensitivity to insulin. A study conducted at the National Institute of Aging at 2003 concluded that mice who fasted regularly compared to mice who consumed the same number of calories had lower levels of glucose and insulin in their blood. This can decrease your risk of getting diabetes. A fasting diet will also help you lose weight which is a risk factor associated with diabetes.

It increases the presence of growth hormone. Growth hormone is made naturally by the pituitary gland and is very important especially in teenagers to enhance their growth. It's become a popular performance-enhancing drug for athletes, but nothing works as good as the real thing! When you're eating too many calories, your body suppresses the secretion of the HGH growth hormone. What fasting does is it signals the glands to secrete HGH and maintain your body mass even if you're not eating for a certain period of time. HGH is involved in lots of body processes to maintain muscle growth and strength and to increase your metabolism so you can lose weight faster.

It increases your mental alertness. It seems counterintuitive — how does not eating make you more alert? But as you're fasting, the body releases norepinephrine which is a hormone that functions to increase the body's energy and focus. Think about how sometimes you're feeling nervous and unable to eat breakfast before a big test? Science proves that actually abstaining from food helps you concentrate better! A research study on mice found that the group that fasted had less short-term memory. It's like how you end up feeling more lazy and lethargic after eating a big meal! You're feeling too full and it dulls your senses. Staying away from food will actually make you more mentally alert.

It can delay aging and help you live longer! A scientific study found that rats that fasted every other day had a more delayed rate of aging and lived 83% longer than their counterpart test group of rats that didn't fast! Another study found that decreasing the amount of calories a test group of mice ate on alternate days by nearly 65%, there were many beneficial health effects that occurred. Those mice had less cardiac issues, lower blood sugar, and had stronger immune systems when it came to fighting infectious diseases. Researchers even believe that fasting can prevent the onset of diseases like multiple sclerosis, Parkinson's, and Alzheimer's! Giving up some food now can give you a longer future! Most people who participate in fasting see that as a big motivator for them.

It can reset your immune system. A study at the University of South Carolina found that fasting anywhere from 2-4 days can regenerate a person's immune system and promote cell-based regeneration. When you're fasting, your white blood cell count goes down. That can sound worrisome but the immune system compensates for it by creating new cells! It triggers cell growth to quickly make up for the shortage. Fasting also makes the cellular process of autophagy occur faster — that's the way the body disposes of any damaged cells. As the immune system is creating new cells, it realizes those damaged cells need to be destroyed. Research shows that the high presence of damaged cells may heighten the chances of getting a neurological disease.

It can increase the effectiveness of chemotherapy. It sounds hard to believe, but research shows that a study on rats found that rats who followed a routine of alternate fasting blocked tumor formation. Another study found that exposing cancer cells to fasting delayed tumor growth and allowed for chemotherapy drugs to be more effective in destroying those cells. More research needs to be conducted on this topic and if you are undergoing chemotherapy, you should speak to your doctor first before embarking on an intermittent fasting diet.

It makes your life easier! We're all busy people and sometimes just finding the time to eat a meal can be difficult! That usually leads to people resorting to fast food and then later regretting that poor meal choice. Instead, skipping that meal altogether and maybe just having a cup of tea or coffee is better for your health in the long run. The caffeine will dull your hunger pangs and get you through the rest of the day. This is much easier to follow than any other diet that has a long list of what foods you can and cannot eat, or make you weigh your food portions and count your calories. There's no headache about making new recipes or shopping for all new ingredients. It's one less meal you need to cook! And knowing all the health benefits you'll gain or some stubborn pounds you'll lose is a great motivator.

Solving the Misconception about Fasting

There are many misconceptions about fasting that people have to break their old notions about. It makes it seem like people who are fasting are jeopardizing their health when in fact, research has proven it has long-term benefits to your overall health. Here are some misconceptions about fasting that we can debunk!

You can't survive without water!

Well, yes, and the very loose "rules" of intermittent fasting is aware of that too! In fact, when you are fasting, you are encouraged to drink lots of water so there is no risk of getting dehydrated. That's necessary for your overall health but especially if you are fasting. If regular water isn't your favorite, then try infused water with fruit or mint leaves or a lemon slice. You want to minimize your calories but make sure you are taking in enough water. You can also have caffeinated beverages like coffee and tea! Caffeine is actually helpful in fooling your body to dull it's sensation to hunger. You want to limit your sugar or cream intake though because those calories add up!

If I don't eat, I'm going to lose my muscle growth!

This is another myth where people seem to believe that if you aren't eating, then you'll lose muscle mass and your muscles will shrink right before your eyes. Not true! After you eat a meal, your body is continuously working to break down your food into carbohydrates to store as energy. You have energy already stored away! When the body has run out of the food you've eaten to use as fuel, then it begins to use the fat molecules it has stored away — NOT muscle tissue! Being without food for just 12-20 hours a day or even a whole day in a fasting on-and-off ritual is not long enough to make you lose muscle mass.

Doesn't skipping breakfast make you gain weight?

Though it's commonly stated that "breakfast is the most important meal of the day," the data shows that it's okay to skip that meal without side effects. People say it'll only increase your craving for food, but a trial study conducted in 2014 showed that between a group of people who ate breakfast and those who didn't, there was no difference in weight gain between the groups after a 16 week trial period. Now, children or teenagers who are in puberty tend to do better in school when they have breakfast in the mornings. That's completely different than an adult who is aware of their health and making voluntary decisions about whether they will skip a few meals or not.

12 hours without food? That's half the day — that's too long!

Here's something that might surprise most people — you're probably already fasting about 12 hours without knowing it! Think of it like this — if you have dinner every night at 7 P.M. and then you have a cup of tea before bed, and then you have breakfast the next morning around 7:30 A.M., you've already fasted for 12 hours! It's all about how you structure your day and fit your schedule to work for your fasting goals. What about 16 hours? It's possible. You sleep in on the weekend and don't have breakfast (or brunch!) until noon — that's 16 hours right there! People who are beginning a ritual of fasting start with a 12 or 16-hour block first and they're sure to fill their time with activities and drink lots of water and caffeine to make the time pass faster!

24 hours without food? A whole day? The human body can't stand that!

Actually... it can! The body is built to withstand many physiological signs of stress so that a person can endure many tough scenarios. Biology shows that the body is meant to use stored fat reserves to create energy if there's a period of no food. Anthropologist says that's how the first societies functioned! Hunters and gatherers would gather what they can, but if there was a period of famine or drought, they would train their bodies to adapt to less and less food. In many primitive societies, that meant the healthy would go without food so the young and elderly could eat. And don't forget all the world religions that fasting rituals in their beliefs. Islam, Judaism, Greek Orthodox Christianity, Buddhism... all include traditions of fasting for healthy, able-bodied individuals. It's a tradition that is millions of years old that people have been partaking in.

Well, I'm an athlete and I don't want fasting to impact my performance negatively.

Another common misconception is that fasting will negatively impact athletes who are in training because they are deprived of energy. Research shows that intermittent fasting does not negatively impact aerobic or anaerobic activity. Just like with the keto diet, all fasting does is encourage your body to begin to burn fat molecules you have stored away instead of carbs. You might feel sluggish in the beginning, but once your body is used to a new energy source, you'll feel your energy return. And fasting encourages you to stay hydrated by drinking plenty of amounts of water! Now, that's intermittent fasting that follows an on-and-off block cycle. If you're fasting for a long period of time without any food intake, that's completely different and can be detrimental to your health.

Is it really true fasting will improve my health in the long run?

Yes, science proves it can! The previous section talks more about the health benefits that fasting provides. Most people just think of fasting as a way to lose weight — which it does do! But it does more than that. Fasting can decrease the chances of getting diabetes, lowers your blood pressure, and even strengthen your heart and lower your cholesterol. This is especially important for people who might have a family history of cardiovascular disease or diabetes.

How to Get Started

If we've got you curious about intermittent fasting and you're wondering how to begin — we have some tips for you! The first few days of following a routine could be tough... just like it's tough to adjust your body to the keto diet. But if you stick to it and surround yourself with motivating factors, you can lose the weight and gain the benefits!

Here are some basic beginner models you can follow!

12/12 Model

This is the beginner's model to follow. It's the easiest because you're probably following it without even knowing it! This model means you are fasting for 12 hours a day continuously then eating for a 12 hour time span. Don't divide it up as day/night but be sure you're watching the time to ensure you're getting 12 hours of time.

Example: You could decide to have dinner every night at 8 P.M. Then be sure to avoid having any late night snacks even though a cup of tea is allowed! This is a great model because it allows you to sleep all night without needing to distract yourself from food. The next morning, don't have breakfast until 8 A.M. You can have a cup of your morning coffee but you want to hold off on breakfast. Unless you work nights or have a very early breakfast, most people are following this model without even knowing it!

16/8 Model

This method follows the model of 16 continuous hours of fasting a day and 8 hours of a continuous eating window. For women, they can change the time blocks to 14-15 hours of fasting instead since women tend to have a lower body mass index than men. A fitness expert, Martin Berkhan, made this method popular as a way to quickly lose weight. If there are only 8 hours of an eating window, you could squeeze in potentially 2 meals and maybe a few healthy snacks to boost your energy. That means eating healthy and avoiding sugary, salty, or processed snacks. People who already skip breakfast or find themselves too busy until brunch time might already be doing this diet. Research shows this model is very helpful in easing indigestion or heartburn before bed. In the morning, you should keep yourself well hydrated and have some morning coffee. Don't forget to keep yourself busy so you're not distracted by your grumbling stomach.

Example: The majorities of people who try this model skip their breakfast and restrict their eating times for the day. That means if you have dinner by 7:00 A.M., then the next morning you shouldn't eat until 12:00 noon. That means you've had 16 hours between meals. This way you can still enjoy a filling lunch and dinner and have some healthy snacks in between.

Now that you have a model to follow, here are some tips to get you started on intermittent fasting!

1. **First, do your research.** Just like with the keto diet, you want to be sure you've done your research about intermittent fasting and understand what you're getting into. You want to know what types of foods you should be eating during your eating window, what model you should be following, and how to track your weight loss. If you have any health issues or taking any medication, you should talk to your doctor first to ensure intermittent fasting is okay for you to try without any risk factors.

2. **Figure out what your goal is.** If you want to have a fasting routine and really stick to it, you're going to need

the right motivation. Do you want to simply lose weight? Do you want to lower your blood pressure or cholesterol? Do you want to see your blood sugar go down so you can eventually reduce your medication? Are you trying to avoid overeating and eating processed or fast food? Find the goal that will motivate you when you are fasting.

3. **Start slow.** Fasting can be challenging especially if you're not used to doing it previously for a religious reason. It can be tough to give up your favorite snacks and meals even for 14 or 15 hours at a time! Don't force yourself into fasting those long chunks of time on day 1. You want to be gentle with yourself and get used to it. First, stop snacking throughout the day so you're cutting back on those calories on food or drinks. Then you can start by skipping one meal like breakfast or sugar. If you are a breakfast person who enjoys having a full plate of things to eat, then skip lunch so you only eat dinner. If you have a big lunch in the middle of the day, skip dinner by keeping yourself busy until bed or just having a cup of tea. Have water instead and force yourself to stay away from those tempting snacks. If you're not a morning person and already skip breakfast, then keep yourself occupied until lunchtime.

It's all about what model works for you and your day. Go slow and follow your body's instincts. When you become more comfortable with getting rid of snacks and skipping a meal, you can try it for a longer block of time. Or you don't have to! Fasting is about what works for you and what you are comfortable with. If you want to stick with the 12/12 model, that works. If you want to attempt the 16/8 model for a few days a week, you can do that too! Stay with what makes you feel healthier and happier.

4. **Keep yourself busy.** Staying away from food can be hard so the best thing you want to do is keep your schedule full! Whether you're occupying yourself with work, reading, spending time with friends (without food involved!), and knitting... whatever it is! Keeping your mind occupied is a great tactic so you're not paying attention to how hungry you are and tempted to just peek into the kitchen. Be aware of gatherings where food is involved and if it makes you break your fast. Choose a place where you won't be tempted and can still be involved.

5. **Stay hydrated.** You should already be drinking enough water but it's even more crucial when it comes to fasting so you don't become dehydrated. Keep a water bottle nearby all day so you can reach for it often and remind yourself to take a few sips. Most doctors say you should have at least 8 glasses of water a day. If you're fasting, you should have about half your body weight in ounces. So for someone weighing 180 pounds, that's about 90 ounces or about 11 8 ounce glasses of water. It sounds like a lot, but if you keep a water bottle handy and remind yourself to fill up throughout the day, you'll have your intake completed. Throw some fruit into your water for more flavors. But be sure you're not using flavored water powder that contains calories.

6. **Get used to other drinks.** You are allowed to have tea or coffee so it's important that when you are fasting you take advantage of these drinks. They will increase your morale when fasting and make your body feel as though you are filling up with calories even though

you're not! Caffeine is proven to actually dull sensations of hunger and triggers the body to release energy it has stored away in fatty acid cells. If you're not a coffee fan, tea is a great alternative. Make sure you're not using cream or sugar though or artificial sweeteners that add calories. Carb-free sweeteners would be the way to go. Calorie-free gum is also a great option to keep you distracted throughout the day.

7. **Get a good night's sleep.** Just like staying hydrated, sleep is important to health in general. But for fasting, even more so! Being well rested can put you in a better mood and ease your irritability or moodiness first thing in the morning. Feeling tired can make you more hungry and wanting to break your fast. After you're done eating, set up your schedule so you're staying away from the temptations in the kitchen and getting to bed earlier. Some extra water or a cup of chamomile tea can help you fall asleep faster.

Conclusion

Thank you for making it through the end of *The #1 Ketogenic Intermittent Fasting Diet Book*! We hope it was informative in helping you learn more about the keto diet and the intermittent fasting lifestyle. We wanted to provide you with information about the health benefits and how the body works to produce results of weight loss if you're correctly following these routines.

It can be overwhelming to follow a diet and learn the rules of what you are and aren't supposed to eat. We wanted to have this book give you a clear picture of what types of foods you can eat on a keto diet — from proteins, vegetables, fruits, alcoholic drinks, and even the limited amount of carbs you are allowed to consume. Counting your calories is important when you begin your diet to ensure you are not overeating. If you are not at the proper ratio of nutrients, your body will not be pushed into the metabolic state of ketosis which is how you lose body fat you have stored away.

With more than 20 meal plans and more than 20 keto-friendly snack recipes, this book is here to help you whip up breakfast, lunch, and dinner to satisfy your cravings and assure you're staying on your diet. You'll be surprised to learn that most of these recipes are easy to make and you probably have all the keto-friendly ingredients in your kitchen. We provide you with many lists to help prepare for the keto diet and what mistakes you want to avoid.

Same goes with intermittent fasting! It can be daunting to start, but we explain the health benefits of fasting — how it can make your heart healthier and even make you live longer! We show you a beginner's model and give you tips on how to get started. Powered with all this information on a healthier lifestyle, you too can lose those stubborn pounds you haven't been able to get rid of and improve your overall health!

www.ingramcontent.com/pod-product-compliance
Lightning Source LLC
Chambersburg PA
CBHW070047230426
43661CB00005B/804